RAPID HEALING
FOODS

Contents

18. Rapid Healing Foods from the Sun for Skin and Hair! 320

1

Rapid Healing Foods Flush Out Poisons for Quick Pain Relief!

Rapid healing foods are really rapid cleansing foods—foods that rid your body of poisons that are the secret cause of many painful ailments—foods that unclog your plumbing, relieve your vital organs of accumulated sludge. When these poisons are flushed out of your body, glorious new health awaits you ... and blessed relief from pain! I call this cleansing power Youth Restorative X.

When these poisons are flushed out of the body, spectacular results are reported, immediate relief can be felt in many cases, like a huge wave of pain lifted and gone forever...heart...liver...gall bladder...kidney...ulcer pain...heartburn...bowel pain...burning urine...sharp head pain...eye, ear and sinus pain...pain in joints...suddenly gone!

Rapid cleansing foods rid your body of poisons—give your entire system a good cleansing. As one of the great exponents of natural healing says, the cause of disease is very nearly always

13

obstruction to the flow of healing forces. Free those blocked channels, and you will have gained health, often immediately!

HOW TO RID YOUR BODY OF POISONS!

What are these poisons that cause so much pain and suffering? They are the germs that cause lung infection with pus ...bladder infection ...boils and running sores. They are the germs that cause putrefaction and decay in the stomach and intestines ...or swelling, inflammation and congestion in various parts of the body. They are the germs that cause a buildup of urinary waste in the bloodstream. They are the excess wastes that cannot be eliminated that turn to solid matter or slime.

This is one of the main causes of growths such as tumors, and ailments that give off thick gooey mucus, like respiratory ailments, and swelling of the mucous membrane of various organs, such as heart, veins, arteries, joints and the lining of the digestive organs— say many doctors—and eliminating this poisonous accumulation can relieve or cure many conditions.

A cleansing diet of certain liquid and natural foods will help rid your body of poisons that have accumulated over the years. When these poisons are flushed out of the body, glorious new health awaits you, say experts ...better breathing ...more vigorous digestion ...pain-free joints ...and added years of health-packed living. Rapid cleansing foods give your entire system (heart, glands, digestion, kidneys, lungs, pancreas, liver) a chance to rest without the additional burden of coping with difficult foods. Rapid cleansing foods rid your body of putrid waste. Partially digested foods that are decaying—and have remained in the system a long time—are washed out! Poisonous germs, solid matter (stones) and thick, gooey mucus are dissolved, broken down and flushed out!

AMAZING QUICK RECOVERIES!

Rapid cleansing foods dissolve, unplug, unclog, clean out and clear debris. They *open* the clogged channels of your body, so that the river of life can flow freely once again! During this rest and relaxation on a diet of cleansing natural food, balance is restored, muscles, glands and organs become strengthened, normal juices flow again and the entire system is energized, invigorated and rejuvenated! In case after case, you'll see how these rapid healing foods are said to—

- Relieve painful backache, leg stiffness, relieve stiff, aching muscles and joints!
- Ward off influenza, asthma, bronchitis, infections, protect you from colds, coughs and respiratory ailments!
- Relieve gas, ulcers, colitis, indigestion, help restore regularity and freedom from pain!
- Help heal stomach and liver disorders, help relieve kidney, bladder and gall bladder problems, strengthen the heart!
- Relieve such problems as baldness, boils, dandruff, eczema, pimples and much more!
- Help relieve headaches, high blood pressure, help improve circulation, relieve hemorrhoids and varicose veins, wash away fatigue poisons from the blood!
- Help melt away extra pounds, automatically!
- Sharpen eyesight, relieve ear problems and much more!

Rapid cleansing foods work primarily by cleansing and purifying the bloodstream, relieving it of toxic poisons and "sludge" that can "clog" the river of life. They push intestinal waste out of the body, break up impacted sludge, melt cholesterol deposits in veins and arteries and help "sweep the body clean"!

KICK THESE HEALTH WRECKERS OUT OF YOUR LIFE!

Millions of people are aging prematurely due to internal toxemia. Toxemia means—simply—poisons in the body. These poisons can secretly cause constipation, clogged bowels, high blood pressure, digestive upset, cramps, overweight, senility, failing mental powers, clogged arteries, painful arthritis, allergies, nervous tension, headaches, failing vision, ringing in the ears, coughs, frequent colds, bronchitis, lung problems, nervous tremors, shortness of breath, fatigue, irritability and vague muscular aches and pains!

These poisons are toxic wastes that come from air, food and poor living habits. They cling to your insides. Some are passed off in breathing, perspiration, urination and bowel movements—but many more remain inside you, clinging to, interfering with and clogging your delicate glands, internal organs, veins and arteries.

They cause what is known as *enervation*, a loss of vigor and failing health. One doctor said that internal poisons were regarded, medically, as "the universal cause of all disease," and recommended internal cleansing as often the only method that brought relief. It is a vicious cycle. Toxemia leads to sluggish body processes—which leads to more toxemia.

ADVANCE WARNINGS!

These poisons give many advance warnings, such as indigestion, poor circulation, sleeplessness and fatigue. They are the hidden cause of many diseases and early aches and pains that have no name. And yet these secret, hidden and dangerous poisons can be seen—to a certain extent—if you look closely. Acne, dandruff, bloodshot eyes, fever, perspiration, yellowish "fat spots" on the skin (cholesterol), gallstones that may be excreted with the stool, kidney stones that may be passed in the urine, warts, arthritic swelling, inflammation of the leg veins (with swelling and congestion, known as phlebitis), puffed eyelids, a gassy bloated feeling, swollen legs and ankles, tartar (discoloration of the teeth), to name just a few, are all solid evidence of poisons in the body.

HOW RAPID HEALING FOODS MAY CURE SPECIFIC AILMENTS!

Astonishing cures are reported with rapid cleansing foods, proving that many serious ailments can be cured quickly, when what to eat and what not to eat are known. Here are the shocking facts:

- When victims of stroke and brain clot were given a certain food—a common vegetable product—that cleans out veins and arteries, sight, hearing and paralyzed arms and legs were returned to normal!

- When a dying lung victim started using a rapid healing food—a common sweet syrup—his lungs became so healthy that doctors refused to believe it was him!

- A common fruit juice can stimulate, purge and empty the gall bladder and has been used to dissolve gallstones! But that's not all. Large kidney stones can be dissolved with it, and the formation of small stones ceases immediately, say doctors!

- At least a half-dozen foods have been found to cleanse the blood of excess sugar. One of them—a common vegetable—has permanently cured diabetics!

- Rapid healing foods have made cataracts melt away! A 90-year-old woman, going blind from cataracts, used two of these foods (common meat and vegetable items). At 94, her cataracts are gone!

- Two common seed oils may relieve MS (multiple sclerosis), muscular dystrophy, cerebral palsy and polyneuritis (paralysis)! Sciatica (leg pain) has been relieved with a common fruit juice, in as little as one day!

- A common vegetable juice has relieved prostate enlargement—even in a case of complete stoppage of urine! The sufferer could urinate freely! It cleared up infection and pus, avoiding surgery!

You'll find out exactly what these foods are, and how to use them, in this book. Rapid cleansing foods available in every supermarket can bring spectacular relief from burns, cure gangrene, ulcerated legs, relieve hay fever, earaches, carbuncles, diabetic dent marks, warts, infections, bedsores, vitiligo, eczema, poison ivy, athlete's foot, stings, heartburn, constipation, diarrhea, colitis, diverticulitis—and may even cure arthritis, rheumatism and gout!

INSTANT PAIN RELIEF FOR SCORES OF AILMENTS

Anything that heals the body is food for the body, because it helps the body heal and regenerate itself. This includes food supplements, massage or anything else that helps sufferers. All are rapid healing, rapid cleansing foods! They can bring instant and immediate relief from the most horrible pains imaginable. Those I tell you about in this book are automatic pain-relieving foods that cured the incurable in case after case!

As mentioned, one of these foods has relieved brain clots and strokes! Paralyzed legs, hands and arms have been cured! Cataracts melted away ...glaucoma symptoms vanished ...hearing returned instantly ...gall stones and kidney stones dissolved and disappeared ...arthritis has been cured ...diabetes actually cured! Heart and lung victims revived and walked away miraculously healed!

Suddenly varicose veins, liver problems, burning urine, burning tongue, headaches, low blood sugar, constipation, colitis, ulcers, burning hemorrhoids, high blood pressure, allergies, skin problems, disappeared in case after case, with these foods. Where one of these foods is eaten, one researcher found men over 90 still able to thread a needle without glasses! Heart disease and cancer were virtually unknown! I'm bursting to tell you the shocking, fully documented facts about these amazing foods—all available without prescription, some from your garden, corner grocery or health food store.

CLEAN OUT VEINS AND ARTERIES!

Take soybeans, for example. Soybeans contain a fatty acid called lecithin that cleans out veins and arteries. One medical doctor says it can save your life. It is the best of all cholesterol reducing agents—and can increase circulation, relieve heart, vein and artery problems, prevent blood clotting and is especially valuable against hardening of the arteries. *Arteriosclerotic plaques are dissolved and removed by this substance*, he says. It has relieved severe angina (heart) pain, reduced cholesterol by 125 points in a little over a month, and in a matter of weeks made extremely high blood pressure drop over 100 points! It has relieved brain clots and strokes, cured paralyzed legs, hands and arms.

- In one case of stroke, brain clot and paralysis, Mrs. A., 83, was too feeble to walk, almost blind, partly deaf, and too weak to feed herself. With this food, in two months, a miracle happened! She walked in to see her doctor under her own power. She was able to see! Because her hearing had returned, they were able to carry on a conversation. She knew she was being healed—she laughed at having cheated death!

- A 65-year-old stroke victim—who'd suffered a brain clot, due to hardening of the arteries—had failing vision, was partly paralyzed, desperate and depressed. With this food, her paralysis gradually disappeared, her vision greatly improved, and she was so radiantly cheerful, she asked: "Doctor, could I go swimming?" "Yes, indeed," he said, "but no diving!"

An 80-year-old woman says that by eating lemon peel, her nausea, dizziness and tendency toward little strokes are virtually cured! A woman with painful varicose veins tried vitamin E, and says: "Three months later . . . No ugly veins bulging on my legs! Even the little 'spider veins' around my ankle were gone!" A woman with phlebitis ulcers tried the same thing and says: "It was like magic . . . The ulcer healed . . . The bulgy veins flattened down to normal . . . Never felt better in my life." Many other foods cleanse or heal the heart, veins and arteries. You'll find full details in Chapter 4.

CLEAN LUNGS!

Here are rapid cleansing foods that clean the lungs, kill the most horrible germs with actual penicillin power, relieve inflammation, lung infections with pus, dissolve mucus and phlegm, cleanse the blood of poisons, relieve asthma, emphysema, bronchitis—clear bronchial tubes—heal lung abscesses, clear up pneumonia congestion in the lungs and much more. Here's how a dying man was saved:

On March 5, 1971, a lung victim was put on the operating table, where doctors found disease so widely spread that it was inoperable. The surgeons sewed him up and declared his case hopeless. On April 5, he heard about a rapid healing food, a common vegetable—and started taking it. By August, x-ray pictures revealed that all signs of disease had disappeared! He is back at work and seems as healthy as ever!

What food wrought this miracle? Asparagus—ordinary canned asparagus, pureed (4 full tablespoonfuls twice daily, morning and evening). Patients have shown dramatic improvement in less than a month. For 25 years, one man reports, he suffered from hay fever every June. Upon hearing of a rapid healing food, honeycomb, he ate some during a severe attack. The hay fever vanished in seconds, and each time it recurred, the same simple remedy banished it! Many other foods have relieved lung and respiratory problems. You'll find full details in Chapter 5.

EYESIGHT AND HEARING RESTORED!

In one reported case, a 60-year-old man suffered from glaucoma. His eyesight was so bad he could only see shadows. On a friend's advice, he began eating three carrots a day, boiled in a quart of water, and drank the water (no seasoning used). In nine days he began to regain his sight. After two months he can see shapes and colors, and identified a friend's Volkswagen parked across the street! In milder cases, eye pressure normalized!

Almost 100 percent cures have been reported for cataracts, using vitamin B-2. Marked healing occurred in 24 to 48 hours, even in advanced cases. Vision cleared and burning, itching, redness and tearing were gone, using 15 milligrams of B-2 daily, nothing else. A doctor reports brilliant results with vitamin E in treating nearsightedness, crossed eyes, cataract and epilepsy. Every patient improved! Epileptic attacks stopped with no sign of return!

Many cases of near-blindness have been helped with vitamin E. Advanced cataracts, even in patients who were totally blind and could not see light, disappeared. A man, suffering nerve-caused blindness, failed to get relief after eight years of treatment. With vitamin E, he could see well enough to dress, feed himself, travel alone and walk through city traffic! A child, 10, born with cataracts on both eyes, was given vitamin E. In a short time, she could see small objects at a distance!

THE DEAF CAN NOW HEAR!

One man discovered a very simple and cheap remedy for bad hearing and ringing in the ears. "My ears would ring so much, and my hearing was very cloudy," he says. "Three years ago I read, 'It is said that a drop of onion juice in the ear is good for bad hearing.' I tried it with wonderful results. Start about three times a week and as your condition improves you may cut down."

One man complained of deafness and a ringing noise in his ear for many years. When he began to eat lots of soybean lecithin every day, suddenly the ringing stopped and his hearing cleared! He is so happy, he plans to keep using this rapid healing food that cleans out fat-encrusted veins and arteries, causing sudden hearing improvement in many cases!

One woman says she uses garlic oil for earaches. "I have seen it work wonders within 10 to 15 minutes of puncturing a garlic oil capsule, pouring it into the ear and stopping it with a little cotton. I have told friends and relatives about how the pain stops soon after, and they all swear by it." Her sister had an inner ear infection. Pain vanished in 15 minutes, with this remedy.

CLEAN LIVER AND GALL BLADDER!

A common tea, chamomile, has long been known to dissolve gallstones. Nicholas Culpepper wrote: "That it is excellent for the stones, appears in this which I have tried—that a stone that hath been taken out of the body of a man, being wrapped in (this tea leaf) will in time dissolve, and in a little time, too."

In one reported case, two gallstones were placed in a glass of this tea. The next day the stones were in four pieces. In five days they were like gravel. In 10 days, they were completely dissolved! A woman says, "I had gallstones. I saw the x-rays, and there were five of various sizes. Through friends...I learned how to get rid of them (with rapid cleansing foods). The gallstones passed on the fourth day. Several years later I had x-rays...and the doctor reported no sign of gallstones."

Here are rapid cleansing foods that cleanse and purify the liver, detoxify putrefactive germs in the bowels to give the liver a rest, stimulate increased blood flow through the liver, relieve a sluggish liver, relieve pain, rejuvenate the liver. One of these foods is said to be the simplest and best treatment when the liver is causing pain. Other foods I tell you about have relieved liver pains in minutes. You'll find full details in Chapter 6.

DIABETICS PERMANENTLY CURED!

Kidney bean pod tea has permanently cured diabetics. Around 1900, a doctor reported that diabetics who had taken this treatment 12 years previously—and stopped using it—stayed cured. Others whose sugar returned were able to find relief again by using it. The length of time involved was three to four weeks, during which a strict diabetic diet was observed.

Years before insulin, many seemingly hopeless cases were cured with this rapid healing food. More recently a lady reported her sugar dropped from 326 to 128 in two weeks, and a kidney stone disappeared, with this tea!

Only the pods are used. They must be fresh. Boil 1 ounce in 4 quarts of water, slowly, for four hours. Filter through fine muslin, cool eight hours, strain again. Take one glassful every two hours. Tea more than 24 hours old causes diarrhea, and ulfiltered tea causes stomach upset. Otherwise, it is reportedly harmless. Other foods have apparently cured diabetes. See details in Chapter 8.

CLEANSE KIDNEYS AND BLADDER!

This same miracle cleansing food—a common tea—has completely relieved kidney blockage of long duration. Bleeding from any part of the urinary system was quickly halted. Stones and gravel were rapidly dissolved, and did not return! Diseases of the bladder and ureter were cured! It drained away pounds of excess fluid—permanently! Many report amazing results!

- **A man with violent kidney stone pains that tormented him constantly for nine years, tried this rapid healing food. "I did not have long to wait for results," he says. "Large masses of uric acid crystals...were excreted...I was soon entirely free from my very great sufferings and have not had any trouble since."**
- **A woman with dropsy (accumulation of fluid) following a valve disease of the heart tried it, after everything else failed. In three weeks, all signs of swelling and dropsy were gone and never returned.**

A popular Thanksgiving Day vegetable is used to clear up burning and scalding urine with infection and pus, soothe inflammation due to gravel or stones, regulate the flow of urine (whether too much or too little) in cases of bladder drip, inability to hold urine, urine retention or stoppage of urine. It seems to heal diseased areas of the kidneys, bladder and urinary passages, and flush out uric acid, toxins and other poisons. A woman whose x-rays showed part of one kidney completely black used it. Later, x-rays showed an entirely clear kidney. Her doctor, surprisingly, said this vegetable was where they got their kidney medicine. The vegetable is corn. The cob and husks are removed. Only the silk is used. Put a handful of the dried brown silk in a stew pan of water, boil for 15 minutes and drink the water. It's as simple as that. It reportedly works wonders in clearing up kidney trouble, a proven remedy.

Large urate stones (stones caused by excessive uric acid) found in the urinary tract can be dissolved with a common fruit, according to the Chief Urologist at a Vienna hospital. He said that such stones have been dissolved by having patients drink the juice of one or two lemons a day. It worked in about 50 percent of all cases of large urate stones. "Where small stones occur chronically, the symptoms as well as the formation of new stones cease immediately," he claimed. For more details on kidney, bladder and urinary problems, see Chapter 7.

ARTHRITIS RAPIDLY RELIEVED!

One drugless practitioner, a doctor of osteopathy, claimed you can *cure* arthritis with rapid cleansing, rapid healing foods. He said that patients would come into his office doubled up with pain and completely hopeless, convinced that nothing could possibly help. Then the amazed look on their faces when the pain disappeared. It didn't matter whether they were old or young …in what part of the body they had arthritis…whether they were still getting around or were bedridden…or how long they had it, 10 days, 10 months, 10 years or longer.

Expect a miracle, he emphasized, because arthritis can be cured! All forms of arthritis! Arthritis of the fingers, shoulders, hips or knees, osteoarthritis, rheumatoid arthritis or any other kind of arthritis. With rapid healing foods, he said, pain and swelling disappear—

almost overnight! Even bone structure can be returned to normal. Results are immediate and spectacular, he said!

This doctor said rapid healing foods offer not only relief, but an end to the condition. Age is no barrier. Legs, hips, back, fingers and knees are healed and cured, he said. With this method, you can expect a miracle of freedom from pain, new freedom of motion and an absolutely pain-free, arthritis-free tomorrow. Complete and permanent cures are possible, pain is relieved right from the start, and aspirins and drugs can be eliminated in a week to 10 days, he stated. As proof, he offered actual x-ray photographs of knee caps unfusing, compressed vertebrae regenerating, bony overgrowth disappearing and returning to normal. These x-rays are positive proof that arthritis *can* and *is* being cured, said this doctor. Seemingly hopeless cases, who were resigned to life in a wheelchair, are now walking and enjoying pain-free, drug-free days once again, he said. Even the agony of weather changes can be a thing of the past!

You, too, may free yourself from the agonies and tortures of arthritis, said this doctor. "I want you to *know* that you can be cured (with astounding speed)," said this doctor!

Rapid cleansing foods, said this doctor, will not harm pre-existing conditions such as gall bladder, ulcer or colitis. Instead, these healing foods will help correct them. "If in the process of curing your arthritis you drop a few other ailments, will you protest?" he asked.

The drugless healing secrets revealed in this book are quite similar to the steps this doctor uses, and are well-known to naturopathic doctors. The one outstanding feature of this method is: no special equipment is needed. It can be used right in your own kitchen, at your own dining table. All you really need is a refrigerator, knife or blender in most cases. All rapid healing foods can be easily obtained, at no extra cost, and perhaps even a cost saving. Other simple steps include aids to elimination (for purification and internal cleansing), and a very few other simple steps. No gadgets or hocus pocus, no bigger and better pills, no expensive therapy or harsh exercises of any kind.

● **There is a rapid healing food I tell about that may bring amazing relief from arthritis—without drugs! All day, all** night relief that seems permanent, in many cases! This fruit is often used in ice cream, cake, candy and desserts! One woman says she started eating it more than 10 years ago. Within a few hours the pain disappeared from her shoulder and arm! The food: fresh cherries!

- Another woman says: "I started eating (this rapid healing food) about a month and a half ago. After about a week, I woke up one morning and felt like a new person . . . swelling was gone and I could bend my fingers completely and painlessly. My wrists and ankles shrank . . . Painful years of suffering . . . were gone. I couldn't believe it."

- Kenneth D., 92, was senile and completely crippled with arthritis. He had to be lifted out of bed and could not feed himself. On a doctor's advice, he was given 1 teaspoonful per day of a rapid healing food. Suddenly he began to perk up! He got out of bed, hobbled into the kitchen and began fixing breakfast! After being senile and crippled for many years, he began to get up every morning—without help. The excruciating pain in his hip no longer bothered him. The only new item in his food or drink was this rapid healing food, concentrated sea water (the kind sold in health food stores that is germ-free), 1 teaspoonful per day!

All over America miracles are happening with rapid healing foods. In cases of arthritis, rheumatism and gout, sufferers claim these foods bring remarkable relief from the agonies of painful arthritic joint inflammation and stiffness, give comforting relief—all-day, all-night relief that seems permanent in many cases—reduce swelling and stop arthritic pain. All enthusiastically agree that rapid healing foods give faster, more effective relief than they ever got before!

HEAL STOMACH AND INTESTINES!

Rapid cleansing foods rid your body of putrid waste. Partially digested foods that are decaying—and have remained in the system a long time—are washed out. Poisonous germs, solid matter and thick, gooey mucus are dissolved, broken down and flushed out. Rapid cleansing foods dissolve, unplug, clean out and clear your stomach and intestines, push intestinal waste out of the body, break up impacted sludge and wash the system clean of many impurities.

- You'll discover a rapid healing food that can cleanse the stomach and intestines of decayed, fetid or putrefying protein wastes that have been only partially digested, with a powerful enzyme. Here is an invaluable aid for feeble digestion, that helps clear up gas, heartburn, diarrhea and the incomplete digestion of foods. It has brought near-miraculous results in cleansing the digestive organs!

- Bleeding ulcers may be healed with certain rapid healing foods. One man who had been in and out of hospitals every week for over a year—doctors were urging the removal of part of his stomach—tried them. They relieved his terrible pain. He forgot all about his ulcer medicine, and in 2 months his ulcers disappeared!

- You'll discover rapid cleansing foods that stimulate normal bowel activity. One of them, for example, is a powerful laxative that cleanses germs of putrefaction in the intestines, and relieves constipation by causing regular wave-like-motions of the intestines. One woman, terribly constipated after reducing 120 lbs, had to strain so hard she thought she'd burst a blood vessel. She tried a rapid cleansing food, and immediately started having normal bowel movements! Others report the same amazing relief!

You'll discover a rapid healing food that has relieved heartburn and ulcers immediately. Another has relieved diverticulitis! Other foods I tell you about relieved hemorrhoids, rectal itching, sores. Another has relieved constipation immediately! A man who had terrible gas pains after having three quarters of his stomach removed, tried a rapid healing food and says: "My gas pains practically disappeared. I feel 100 percent better!" Another food has relieved cramps, spasms and colitis, and stopped diarrhea immediately! It gave permanent relief in many cases, even in the extreme diarrhea of dysentery! Poisons in the system are the only reason for degeneration of any kind. Rapid healing, rapid cleansing foods rid your body of poisons— give your entire system a good cleaning. One of them, for example, is the most powerful antibiotic known in food, with actual penicillin power! The total effect is that these foods cleanse and heal!

DOCTOR'S NEW "INSTANT YOUTH" SECRET!

It is the accumulation of poisons in the lungs, the blood-steam, the intestines and various organs of the body that is the most common cause of pain, say drugless doctors. To eliminate uric acid, toxins and other body poisons, these doctors recommend internal cleansing with pain-relieving, healing, rapid cleansing foods that wash the system clean of all impurities.

Automatic pain relief and the cure of specific ailments follows when the body is cleansed of its impurities, say leading experts. In 1911, Dr. Alexis Carrel proved the value of complete cleansing by placing the cells of a chicken heart in a solution containing everything needed for life, cleaning them completely every two days. He kept the unborn chicken heart alive and beating for 30 years!

Scientifically, there is no reason in the world why you cannot keep your heart, glands, digestion and all vital organs in perfect working order, and live a hearty, vigorous life filled to the brim with strength, joy and radiant good health—until you are well over 100—with this secret, discovered by a Nobel Prize winner, for the heart muscles were still beating when the experiment ended, and there is no telling how long they would have continued to do so!

YOU'LL SEE THE RESULTS AND FEEL THE RESULTS ALMOST OVERNIGHT!

The cleansing and nutrition secret, which Dr. Carrel discovered—and which rapid cleansing foods accomplish so well—is one that doctors have been whispering the praises of for years. It is the secret of youthful looks and vigorous long life that millions the world over have been clamoring to learn. They pursue this goal every day in expensive health clubs, health spas and beauty salons—without any hope of ever achieving it because they do not know this secret. But you will! With it, you can restore your youthful health and appearance! Rapid cleansing foods can work wonders in your life, keep you bright and cheerful, ward off many diseases and may even darken prematurely gray hair!

Biologically, there is no reason why you should grow old! Age is not a matter of time. People age and dry up simply because their bodies are bathing in poisons— wastes are not fully carried out by the blood, so that fresh oxygen and nutrients can be carried in.

When circulation is reduced or cut off or made less effective in any way, there is an actual "drying out" tendency of the cells of the body—like leaves dying on a vine—and it is this drying out that causes skin to wrinkle, bones to become brittle and hair to lose its color, and fall out.

FOOL THE CALENDAR!

Why let youth slip through your fingers when medical science has proven beyond the shadow of a doubt that you can hold off aging for 10, 20, 30 years or more—and actually reverse the aging process, as Dr. Benjamin Frank has shown in his experiments with nucleic acids, present in many of these power-packed foods!

Now you can be brisk, active and youthful at an age when others are gray and broken! You can have abounding vitality, and the abundant vigor and energy that go with it, say leading experts. Now you may cheat time of 20 or 30 years! Nature will amaze you as she restores your body in a fraction of the time it took to age. You will feel decades younger, and this can happen almost overnight, say experts!

Even in advanced age you can be healthy and your appearance can fool the calendar. With these pain-relieving foods, you can actually feel the years roll back as every tiny cell in your body fills out and grows young and firm again. Headaches, tired blood, leg congestion, varicose veins and impotence caused by blood-starved sex cells, can become a thing of the past!

CELL TISSUE REJUVENATION!

Perhaps you cannot cleanse your body of every poison (although I firmly believe that nothing is incurable), but you *can* drastically reduce the effect of years of accumulated waste from junk foods, pollution, poor living habits, with these amazing rapid healing foods . . . surround every tiny cell with all the life-giving elements it needs . . . and add, perhaps, up to 30 health-packed years to your life, starting now, with foods so powerful they seem like bionic healing foods!

The secret ingredient in all these foods is their natural cleansing power. I call this cleansing power Youth Restorative X. All rapid cleansing, rapid healing foods contain Youth Restorative X. And anything that heals the body is food for the body, because it helps the body regenerate itself!

You can undergo complete and actual cell-tissue rejuvenation, with rapid healing foods. You will not only look younger and feel younger, you will actually be younger. For example, alternate muscle tensing and relaxation is nature's way of flushing out poisons from the system. The cleansing power this provides is, indeed, rapid healing, rapid cleansing food for the body. Spectacular results are reported! Now re-discovered after nearly a century—Youth Restorative X, the secret that may actually make you young again, the miracle rejuvenation secret that shows you how men and women in ther 50s, 60s, 70s, and even 80s were able to look and feel half their age, how a man in his seventh decade claimed it did all this and more. His name was Anton L.

MIRACLE YOUTH RESTORATIVE X

In an amazing narrative, written around the turn of the century, Anton L., at 65, claimed to have discovered a miracle youth restorative that gave him the appearance of a man half his age! Specifically, he claimed—

It restored his sight, his hair—erased his wrinkles, and gave his skin the smooth appearance of youth! It made his rheumatism vanish, restored his liver, healed his stomach ulcers and varicose veins, reversed his hardening of the arteries, without surgery—and all without pills or potions!

He called it Youth Restorative X, and claimed that anyone could use it, quickly and easily, to flush age-causing poisons out of the body. He cited many cases to prove that Youth Restorative X may actually make you young again.

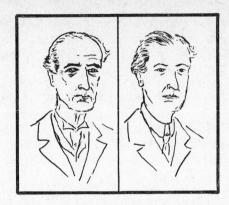

MAN WHO GREW YOUNG AT 65 CLAIMS DISCOVERY OF YOUTH RESTORATIVE X

Anton's story is made even more believable by the fact that he had nothing to sell. At 60, he suffered a complete physical breakdown, and was bedridden for many weeks. It gave him time to think, and after much research he hit upon this method of using a rapid cleansing food, exercise—to flush out poisons—which he said are the cause of old age. In writing of the amazing change in his appearance, he said:

> "At 60, I was physically an old man...I was then balding, my thin hair streaked with gray, with loose-hanging jowls and puffy bags under my eyes. I was nearly blind, my pulse was irregular, I had liver problems, ulcers, weak lungs, varicose veins and hardening of the arteries, with acid rheumatism adding its agonies. I was an old man and looked it."

With this simple method, so remarkable was his recovery that at 65 he looked to be 35 or 40, and felt it. Yet he had solid proof of his age, in the form of legal documents, army discharge papers, testimonials from reputable doctors and remarkable before and after photos. He retained his vigorous good looks for nearly 100 years!

THE FIRST PROVEN CASE OF ACTUAL REJUVENATION!

With Youth Restorative X, in a matter of weeks, he started growing younger. When he was 65, his family doctor reported:

"At this time I find a great change in Anton L.'s appearance. He really seems rejuvenated. The hair has become luxuriant. No indication of baldness. The skin is smooth, no longer loose and hanging...face smooth. He has the appearance of a very young man of 35 or 40. The lines which formerly existed have disappeared!"

The doctor continued: "Heart sound, no palpitation or irregularity of pulse, digestion good, liver sound, ulcers healed, lungs healthy, no indication of varicose vein or hardening of the arteries, eyes normal, joints limber, he seems very alert, no trace of senility, his mind is sharp and clear. He says he has devised a method that eliminates dead or clogging material from the body."

CLAIMS EYESIGHT RESTORED!

For many years, Anton was plagued with poor vision. Long hours of work, as a bookkeeper, had ruined his eyes, until finally he was nearly blind. "The light failed," as he put it. He recovered partially by resting completely, and then suffered a relapse. He was unable to read, strong light was painful to his eyes and he stumbled about pathetically...

Yet with this secret, at 65, his sight improved so much he was able to see without glasses, do extensive reading and research and his eyes were no longer painful. "This great improvement in my sight," he wrote, "is certainly directly due to this secret."

He claimed this method has a wonderfully invigorating effect upon the eyes and will surely improve the sight. The reason for this is that it draws the blood to the eyes, and increases their vitality by enabling them to secure more and better nourishment. It also stimulates the nerve structures of the eyes.

DARKENS AND RESTORES HAIR!

At 60, Anton was quite bald, and what little hair he had was thin and streaked with gray. At 65, his doctor noted: "The hair has become luxuriant. No indication of baldness." With this method, Anton claimed:

New healthy hairs will spring up in place of dead ones, often from the same root! Wherever life remains in the follicles, new hairs will sprout, he said! Anton found it possible to stimulate the gland that produces hair color by certain simple hand movements. As a result, his hair became much darker!

With this method, Anton claimed, it is possible to actually restore hair to its original color! Here are the methods by which he claimed hair loss can be arrested (full details in Chapter 16)—

- A common food that is a valuable tonic for both hair and scalp, as it accelerates the circulation. This natural substance is far more powerful than any medicinal "hair invigorator" yet invented, he says!

- A simple method that could help thousands save their hair …what to do for an itchy scalp…how to relieve dandruff problems…a simple method used in certain countries where baldness is almost unknown!

- A simple lotion you can make and use that will rid you of any germs or disease on the scalp. This excellent tonic, he said, is harmless and superior to any advertised expensive hair tonic or germicide!

"If life still remains in the roots of the hair a healthy growth will usually result," said Anton. "This method is easy, inexpensive and effective, and can actually restore your hair."

MAKING OLD FACES YOUNG!

A picture of Anton, at 60, shows under the chin, the loose-hanging skin of age. After using this method—in a few weeks—the loose folds disappeared, and five years later, they were still gone.

With Youth Restorative X, he claimed, it is really very easy to rejuvenate the throat and face. Even after middle age, he said, wrinkles will disappear, and the smoothness of youth will be regained rapidly!

You don't need expensive plastic surgery. You can give yourself a permanent natural face-lift. It involves no expense, is painless and very effective. All you need are the tips of your fingers and the palms of your hands. Any disfiguring bags will disappear. If the throat is too fat and full, if you have a double-chin, this method will speedily reduce it, he said.

CLAIMS RHEUMATISM DISAPPEARED!

At 60, Anton complained of creaking, painful bones and joints. He cried out in pain, and resolved to find a way to make them flexible once again. With Youth Restorative X, in a short time all signs of rheumatism disappeared!

This method, he claimed, may even effect a cure not possible with drugs. If there is any tendency to rheumatic pains in the limbs—where deposits of uric acid frequently occur—this method will relieve it by dislodging such deposits.

"Uric acid is the basic cause of rheumatism," said Anton. "It accumulates in the system from wrong foods, faster than the kidneys can eliminate it, and forms into crystals, like so many splinters, which settle in muscles and joints. Youth Restorative X compels these hardened 'stones' to break up, dissolve and be eliminated by the natural excretions of the body. It is the simplest, easiest and most effective way to relieve acute rheumatic pain."

SLUGGISH LIVER RELIEVED!

For 30 years, Anton complained of chronic indigestion, a belching bitter taste, pains on the right side, gas, headache, dizziness, nausea, foul breath, constipation, chills, perspiration, drowsiness after meals and heart palpitations, all common symptoms of liver and gall bladder problems.

With this secret, said Anton, all symptoms of a sluggish liver disappeared. Youth Restorative X will do wonders in relieving liver complaint, and stimulating a sluggish liver, he claimed. It is safe and harmless, and only benefit will result, he said.

Anton used a simple hand motion on the liver, done in bed, in the morning, when the stomach is empty. "The next time your liver is sluggish," he said, "try my plan and you will not regret it. It can be done under the most comfortable conditions. It really works. I never take any pills or potions any more."

STOMACH ULCERS, CONSTIPATION, AND OTHER DIGESTIVE DISORDERS RELIEVED!

It is not surprising that Anton suffered from both ulcers and rheumatism, as both are symptoms of an acid condition pervading the entire body. The cause of his trouble was the way he ate, but he never changed his eating habits. Youth Restorative X relieved his trouble entirely.

Thanks to this method, all his digestive problems disappeared. "I eat whatever I like, and lots of it," he said. Nearing 100, he still boasted a ravenous appetite, due to this rejuvenation method which stimulates all organs, both digestive and glandular.

"It is Nature's simplest remedy for stomach upset," said Anton, "and can help you avoid heartburn, gas, cramps and other symptoms of indigestion. It is fast, easy, and totally without cost. I was never a healthy man until I discovered this secret—and have never taken any medicines since."

- You'll discover a simple food you can take, 15 minutes before breakfast, that is a good remedy for constipation ... how to keep the colon or lower bowel clean ... the one simple thing most of us do that is the cause of 85% of digestive disorders, Anton said.

- This method cleanses the colon without the slightest physical effort, in about 15 minutes. "It is the simplest and most effective method, and is an important factor in my system of physical rejuvenation. I strongly advise it be used," he said.

- The importance of keeping this large intestine clear of obstruction is easily apparent. If anything is allowed to become clogged with fecal matter, as in the case of constipation, it becomes the incubating ground of disease-breeding germs, and the source of all manner of diseases and complications, which would not occur if it were kept properly clean, say many experts.

Youth Restorative X greatly assists the stomach, intestines, liver, kidneys and all organs of elimination in expelling noxious waste and clogging matter, which causes decay of vital organs. It has a beneficial effect on the entire system, calms the nerves and is a sure cure for insomnia. In a very short time after using it, you will see that digestion and elimination are greatly improved, said Anton.

LUNG PROBLEMS RELIEVED!

Anton claimed this method healed his lungs, relieved his asthma and bronchitis, and was a sure cure for colds, relieving them almost overnight, and cleared up sinus problems, even early pneumonia. Anton wrote: "My mother died of consumption at 38. I inherited her weak lungs, and throughout my sickly, feeble childhood, I suffered from asthma and bronchitis. Everyone said I would surely go as my mother did.

"Yet today at 65, I am hale and hearty. I have come back from a gasping, wheezing invalid, plagued with respiratory ailments to one who is absolutely free from coughs, colds or any lung weakness. I strongly urge that you use this method for lung health."

"With Youth Restorative X, you need not fear pulmonary diseases. By this lung strengthening method, I have increased my chest expansion and doubled my lung capacity. After using this secret myself, I can confidently state that only good will result."

HOW TO CURE A COLD!

Anton L. claimed he had a sure cure for colds, that relieved them quickly—almost overnight! As a young man with weak lungs and a tendency to respiratory ailments, he dreaded catching cold. It always meant a long period of illness, for he recovered very slowly from such attacks. On one occasion, when he caught an "awful cold," he discovered how to get rid of it.

A doctor who did not believe in medicines advised him to use a simple remedy, and guaranteed a speedy recovery with this method. "I took his advice. The results were exactly as he had stated," said Anton. "In two days, I was entirely recovered, without any trace of a bad cold!"

"It was amazing," he says, "because I fully expected a two-week siege, and here I was, completely well. And this is how I have cured my bad colds ever since for the past 40 years. The proven fact is, this method does cure colds quickly, without expensive drugs. It is one of the reasons why my lungs are so healthy today, at 65." With this quick and easy cure for "bad colds" the clogging rubbish is burned up or eliminated from the body and glandular structures. It also clears up serious sinus problems quickly. And in the early stages of pneumonia, a cure is almost certain, said Anton.

VARICOSE VEINS HEALED!

In varicose veins, a steady upright position produces stagnation of blood in the legs, and pressure on veins, which enlarge. This cannot be cured by lotions or medicines. Surgery is expensive and painful. Temporary relief can be obtained with an elastic stocking, but the trouble returns. The first sign of trouble is a dull, aching pain. The vein becomes much larger, knotted and distended, and sometimes bursts.

Anton claimed this method is a sure cure in any ordinary case. At 40, he developed a painful, bulging varicose vein which annoyed him for the next 20 years. It was always annoying, and threatened to ulcerate or form a clot. For years, he wore an elastic stocking.

"Relief is obtained by this method. It will relieve the congestion, and restore the distorted venous valves to their proper position, when the trouble will disappear. It is a simple, easy and effective remedy for this very annoying affliction," said Anton. All you need are the palms of your hands, while relaxing in bed. At 65, Anton's legs were so healthy, he ran a mile in 7:50 to prove it, without any distress, which he could not do at age 40!

(Anton did this only for demonstration purposes. "I do not approve of such strenuous effort after middle age," he said, "but was willing to give the exhibition to show the effects of this method. The pulsation of my heart returned so quickly to normal that a very able doctor declared I am as fit as a young man half my age.")

HOW TO LOSE WEIGHT RAPIDLY BY EATING MORE WITH YOUTH RESTORATIVE X

Ordinary diets often produce a weakened condition which affects the heart, said Anton. They do not remove fat where you want it, and involve a great deal of self-denial. Anton *overate*, and yet he remained slender!

"I eat whatever I like, and lots of it," he said! And yet he claimed this method will melt off pounds faster than anything else in the world. No calorie counting or willpower is needed. "This method is the surest, easiest and safest method of losing fat," he said. His own "spare tire" disappeared, and so will yours, he emphasized!

Youth Restorative X, he said, has the same effect on fat as it has on clogging, age-causing debris in the body—it causes fat to be expelled from the body. The fat is loosened, burned up and carried off by the process of excretion. With this method, there is an increased flow of blood to fatty areas, bringing oxygen. As oxygen comes in contact with the fatty deposit, the fat is burned up, said Anton. It is a very effective way of attacking unwanted fat deposits, and can be done most easily and effectively while lying in bed!

HARDENING OF THE ARTERIES REVERSED!

Anton claimed his secret was a major breakthrough in reversing hardening of the arteries, which he said is the principal cause of "old age." As we advance in years, he said, there is a clogging up of the arteries by chalky deposits. As technically described, it is arteriosclerosis, "a filling up and hardening of the arteries."

Think of the arteries as a network of tubes, carrying blood to the organs. When these tubes become clogged, the blood supply diminishes. Organs deteriorate. That is old age. The blood supply to the brain becomes less and less, for example, and the vigorous brain of middle life gives way to loss of memory, confusion and general imbecility of old age.

Youth Restorative X eliminates those clogging deposits and prevents their return, said Anton. With free circulation restored, the body again becomes youthful. Anton's sudden return to health at 60, and his excellent physical condition at 65, is the best proof of these statements.

MIRACLE YOUTH RESTORATIVE X CLEANS OUT ARTERIES!

Youth Restorative X opens clogged arteries, whether the largest tube in the system or the most microscopic capillary, said Anton. It cannot be accomplished by any other means, all medical preparations, however highly recommended, to the contrary, said Anton. Experts have stated:

> If the arteries can be kept clear of this clogging sludge, they will remain open and youthfully flexible, the heart will pump blood through them without effort, while all the vital organs, receiving a generous blood supply, will regain their vigor, and the body will present the appearance of youth, even at an advanced age.

At 60, Anton was feeble with age, and a general hardening of the arteries. In a matter of weeks, this condition was reversed, and he was young again at 65!

FLUSHES POISONS OUT OF THE BODY!

"If this clogging waste matter can be eliminated, then the conditions of youth will return," said Anton. Youth Restorative X forces out from the body any waste matter which may have deposited into the venous and glandular system, and it is then carried off by the ordinary bodily excretions.

> Youth Restorative X flushes out that rust or clogging debris, and then you feel "limbered up" and "good as new" again. In a matter of minutes, you experience a healthy glow and wide-awake feeling. It is a proven way to physical rejuvenation, and works equally well for men or women!

If the human body is kept free from worn-out tissue, dead cells or other clogging matter, it will not exhibit what we know as "the signs of age" to a period long past what we now think to be the limit of youth, said Anton. These poisons can be forced out of the body, actually "pumped" out, he said. That is the secret of rejuvenation.

THOUSANDS HELPED BY THIS AMAZING SECRET!

Anton L. succeeded in rejuvenating his old body to a degree far beyond that which he had supposed possible. "As I do not differ from other human beings in my physical structure, what has been possible in my case is just as possible in yours." Anton L. gave his step-by-step method to many people. Thousands tried it.

Do you think you are too old? Remember, Anton L. began his experiment in rejuvenation at 60, an age when many think that such dramatic results are impossible to attain. Thousands who tried Youth Restorative X, age 60-75, obtained the same results in a very short time.

"I feel absolutely certain that what I have done you can do. You will probably succeed far more rapidly than I have," he said. "I had to pioneer my own way. And now, in my 65th year, I present the appearance of a man little more than half my age. What I accomplished is possible to almost anyone."

"WHAT I ACCOMPLISHED IS POSSIBLE TO ALMOST ANYONE!"

Anton's success in regaining, at 65, the condition of youthful health was so remarkable that it was absolutely convincing. The annals of medicine cannot show any case in which, by the use of drugs, such results have been obtained.

When at 60, Anton found he was certainly becoming younger, he thoroughly investigated his family and its branches for nearly 200 years. The results of that search were that he was not descended from a long-lived family. Yet he lived to nearly 100 with Youth Restorative X!

"The method by which I have made this success has the advantage of being entirely without cost," he stressed. All you need are a few simple instructions—nothing else. There are no scientific names to puzzle you. "What has been possible in my case is, most probably, just as possible in yours," he said.

OVERCOME THE BARRIER OF TIME!

Youth Restorative X, if used faithfully, will result in improved circulation, healthy glandular activity and will materially prolong your life, says this expert. It expels all clogging debris—rids the body of all poisons, he said. Give nature a chance. Try it. It is the safe way, the easy way, the natural and inexpensive way to cleanse and revitalize the body. "I am positive you will succeed," said Anton. Read on for full details.

DOCUMENTED PROOF THAT RAPID HEALING FOODS WORK!

This book is going to shock and astound you because, reportedly, rapid healing foods can bring cures to diseases and injuries which many doctors consider virtually incurable. With these foods, countless thousands cured themselves of seemingly hopeless ailments—even avoiding surgery—when doctors said it couldn't be done!

I am not a writer of fiction, and the information contained in this book is all based on documented facts. My files are filled with cases that read like miracles. With rapid healing foods many users report it was as if they pushed a magic button to instant pain relief!

Described here are tough, resistant, hard-to-heal conditions deemed incurable by doctors—cases where all else failed—that were completely and permanently cured, or apparently abated, with no sign of return. One drugless doctor claims that you can heal all but the most grievous illnesses entirely by yourself, without drugs, without cost, without painful treatments and, except in rare instances, entirely without the services of a doctor. With rapid healing foods, he says, in a mere single week you may discover that ailments you were resigned to enduring all your life have gone, fairly evaporated away!

Another drugless healer claims you have the power this very moment to experience a complete cure for many diseases, no matter how horrible their reputation, and quickly end all pain and suffering. That goes for many ailments associated with great pain, like ulcers, arthritis, heart ailments and many more. I mean to say that drugless healers (some medical doctors, too) report that you can experience absolute relief, often without medicines or surgery. In fact, rapid healing foods are reported 100 percent successful in curing many ailments, used as directed. Some healers claim there is no disease or injury you cannot heal this way, that even the toughest illness can be cured, and that this secret can restore you to perfect health. Results are amazingly fast, bringing relief often in a matter of seconds.

THE SECRET OF PERFECT HEALTH AND COMPLETE FREEDOM FROM DISEASE

A famous doctor once stated that disease of the body is a result always of the body's inability to keep itself clear of its own accumulated debris. Drain the body of its poisons, feed it properly and miracles of healing happen!

With this secret, which I call Youth Restorative X, diseases of all kinds actually disappear, and we are rewarded with the highest degree of natural immunity, said this doctor. Health and long life are virtually guaranteed!

We have then safeguarded all functions; we have reduced the liability of infection to practically zero; we have prevented the annoying daily fatigue from which so many suffer; we have guaranteed ourselves against disease; we have postponed old age to some time in the indefinite future, he claimed.

Age is not a matter of years, said this doctor, but is due rather to the retention of acid waste matter. Certain foods are acid-forming, while others are alkaline or base-forming. We need four times as much of these alkaline foods, for these quickly neutralize acids as they form. Rapid healing, rapid cleansing foods are almost invariably alkaline. They are the secret of perfect health and complete freedom from disease. Along with this, internal cleansing plays an important part in this method of rejuvenation. Spectacular results were reported by this doctor:

- Pneumonia, erysipelas, influenza, acute arthritis, colitis, hay fever, all subside when the body is flushed or cleansed of poisons, with rapid healing foods, he said!
- Many cases of nephritis, unable to walk due to weakness, unable to lie down because of shortness of breath, after

three days of a cleansing diet, can lie down flat to sleep and even take walks with enjoyment. Results are rapid and astonishing, said this doctor!

- True angina (heart pain), whether from degenerative changes in the heart muscle or from embolism of the coronary artery, will generally lose all pain on exertion after three days of a cleansing diet, and go on to complete relief, even returning to active exercise, golf, even tennis, with no trace of heart weakness, he said!

- Almost every case of arthritis will respond to treatment, said this doctor. Complete recovery is the rule, not the exception!

- Many a case of gastric or duodenal ulcer responds at once, the very first day of a rapid healing diet bringing grateful relief. Complete and permanent cures are possible in nearly all cases, he said!

- Out of 109 cases of progressive pernicious or primary anemia, complete and permanent cures were obtained in all but eight cases with this method!

- Seemingly hopeless cases of asthma recover quickly with this method, he said—especially the chronic, spasmodic type who has been everywhere, tried everything, seen all the best specialists and been told nothing can be done except to live with it. In as little as three days there is marked, and often permanent, relief that seems almost unbelievable, he claimed!

- Every case of colitis recovers with this method of ridding the body of its toxic mass of putrefying, fermenting waste that has been retained too long, said this doctor.

- Many experienced virtual immunity from colds!

Of all the thousands of cases treated with this method, in 26 years of practice, nearly all regained their health, said this doctor.

IMPORTANT NOTICE
TO READERS OF THIS BOOK!

All recognized authorities state that self-medication is inadvisable, without a doctor's approval. You are advised to seek a doctor's advice immediately, for any condition which has been bothering you. This book is a reference work only, and its directions are not to be considered prescriptions for any ailment you may have. Since I am neither a physician, consultant, nor medical practitioner, I do not diagnose or prescribe. I only report what others have done, and what they have claimed for the methods described herein. Nor does this book reflect the majority opinions among doctors. The use of ordinary non-prescription foods as medicine is controversial. Some doctors praise them highly, and recommend them to everyone. They are considered minority unorthodox practitioners.

AMAZING HOME REMEDIES!

So, what we have here are amazing home remedies you've probably never heard of before—simple things that you can do yourself, at home, at little or no cost, with your doctor's approval—to relieve aches and pains all over the body.

Many of these home treatments may be labeled "old wives" tales by the medical profession—such as raw vegetable juices, herbal tonics, massage or the simplest use of ordinary tap water—but they have helped many seemingly hopeless cases, where all else failed, even avoiding surgery!

While not a substitute for qualified medical care—always obtain your doctor's permission before using—they may help you quickly when needed. Some of these remedies are jealously guarded professional secrets. Some are relatively new. Some are thousand of years old. All are rapid healing foods for relief of grievous ailments—available everywhere without prescription, some from your garden, corner grocery or health food store. No one knows exactly why they work. They just do. You will often be astounded at the results, just as I have in my many years as a health researcher and medical research reporter.

In writing this book, I have done considerable research. All claims and experiences are the actual reports of people who have used these methods. My studies ranged from the inception of the nature cure movement in the early 1900s to the present date. Various source materials were used, ranging from recent medical reports to books published within the last year or so. Unless otherwise indicated, all unidentified doctor quotes are from books written in the 20s and 30s. My studies show that the basic principles of drugless healing have not changed over the years, and I believe they are just as valid today as when originally written.

2

Rapid Healing Foods for Stomach and Intestines!

Indigestion means, literally, the absence of digestion. Usually it results from incorrect food combinations. It occurs chiefly in the stomach, but its effects spill over into the intestines, causing poisonous gas, toxins and discomfort. One medical doctor tells us that:

"If each meal consists of correctly combined foods it is safe to say that indigestion, as we understand the term, would vanish; likewise, much irritability of temper, and much or all physical fatigue!

"If right foods are selected, if they are properly combined, there will be no indigestion, and if no indigestion then no constipation," he says. We should then understand how foods should be selected and combined.

FOODS THAT MAKE OR BREAK YOU!

It is strange when you think of it, that while 90 percent of all natural foods are alkaline, most people live on the 10 percent of foods that are acid-forming. Eat acid-forming foods, and you pay the price in misery and suffering. The foods that make us are largely alkaline. They are rapid healing, rapid cleansing foods that can almost immediately improve your health!

This is best illustrated by the following case, reported by an osteopathic doctor, specializing in eye problems. "One case in particular which I remember was a lady who had lost her sight. Upon questioning her, I found that before losing her sight she had a nervous breakdown. She insisted that she was well fed. When asked what she considered good food, she gave me the following list.

Foods That Break You:

1. whole wheat bread
2. rolled oats
3. cream and sugar
4. roast meats
5. cooked vegetables
6. fresh boiled eggs
7. fresh cured ham
8. butter and milk
9. cocoa and chocolate
10. tea, coffee, dessert

"After she lost her sight, the surgeons decided that it was a case of brain tumor. However, after opening her skull, they found no tumor, and they were very much at a loss to understand why she had lost her sight. When she came to me she had been blind for a year and three months. I was her last hope. Upon examination, we found her to be anemic, troubled with chronic constipation and very nervous. After explaining to her that we would undoubtedly find her intestinal tract loaded with dead mucus, which would have to be removed before her nervous system could be quieted (and that) we would have to give her nothing but the cleansing foods to dispose of the toxic substances, she objected . . . She could not understand how it would be possible for her to live even for a few days on the cleansing foods which I suggested. Among the cleansing foods recommended to her were:

Foods That Make You:

1. pineapple	6. oranges
2. blackberries	7. pears
3. strawberries	8. honey for sweetening (sparingly, but
4. grapefruit	not with oranges or grapefruit)
5. tangerines	

"After she had tried the above diet for three days, she began to see flashes of light, although she had lost some weight and was very weak. The fact that these foods had helped Nature to purify her bloodstream was very evident; she was resting better and became keenly interested in (rapid healing foods). Then we gave her a more substantial diet consisting of celery, radishes, lettuce, greens, coleslaw, young green onions, watercress, spinach, tomatoes, asparagus and a small quantity of whole wheat bread."

AN ASTONISHING CURE!

"These foods, being high in iron, mineral salts and vitamins, improved her condition very rapidly. We allowed her to have only a very few meats; chicken, lamb, veal, fish and eggs— but whenever we gave her a small quantity of these foods, we insisted that with them she have either a large fruit salad containing not more than three fresh fruits, or a large vegetable salad, consisting of not more than three or four fresh raw vegetables. However, fresh fruits and fresh vegetables were not allowed at the same meal. She was instructed to eat fresh fruits whenever she became hungry, regardless of the time of day."

In less than three weeks, she regained much of her vision. She was surprised, while being led to the doctor's office, to notice that she was being steered too near the curbing. On another occasion, she stepped around a small pool of water. It soon became possible for her to see large objects.

"She enjoyed her sleep and her food, and life became more bearable," says this doctor, adding that if she had eaten proper foods, she would never have lost her sight in the first place. "This is so simple and clear to me," he says, "that I many times wonder why people insist on eating foods that have no value."

YOU ARE WHAT YOU EAT!

Foods can literally make or break you. There are foods that produce health—and others that weaken the body. Even healthful foods can be ruined by cooking or bad food combinations. In either case, the body is deprived of their food value, and instead of helping you, these foods become a burden to the digestive system, producing poisons or toxins that can harm you.

Since the human race learned to cook foods, thus demineralizing and devitalizing it, we have produced over 2,400 diseases not found among animals. We also eat for entertainment, thus over-loading our already congested bodies. We spice and season our food to stimulate our appetite.

Appetizers stimulate the mucous lining of the stomach and intestines, causing these organs to secrete large amounts of digestive juices, leaving them depleted and incapable of acting upon natural food when it is received.

HEALTHFUL FOOD COMBINATIONS!

People who eat anything and everything at the same meal, sooner or later, will suffer from headache, sour stomach, gallstones and many other conditions which are caused by wrong food combinations. For example, fruits require not more than one hour for digestion. They should not be eaten at the same meal with fresh vegetables, which require four hours for digestion. One retards the digestion of the other, which gives the body much unnecessary work.

Many people use sugar with fruit. This causes fruit to ferment. Then they are surprised when they develop gas and heartburn. Lower forms of animal life do not require antacids. Neither are they subject to ulcers, colitis, constipation or diarrhea under normal conditions. When they are captured, their stomach and intestines are healthy, free from decay and disease, because they have been eating natural foods containing enzymes and other elements needed for perfect health. Human beings must boil, fry, stew or bake their food until the enzymes, vitamins and other essential elements are destroyed. Then we wonder why we have gas, heartburn, ulcers, constipation and diarrhea.

FOODS THAT MAKE YOU!

The following is a list of foods that contain real food value, in short, the foods that make you. They are rapid healing foods for stomach and intestines:

Oranges	Pineapple	Prunes, dried
Pears (fresh)	Dates	Apricots, fresh
Persimmons	Grapes	or dried
Tangerines	Currants	Peaches
Grapefruits	Loganberries	Raspberries
Limes	Apples	Figs, fresh
Blackberries	Raisins	or dried
Strawberries	Plums	Watermelon
Lemons	Cherries	Cantaloupe

Remember, fresh fruits are first choice. Sun-dried fruits are second choice. Canned fruits are third choice. Canned fruits should be omitted from the diet when it is possible to obtain fresh. Canned pineapple and canned grapefuit are the exceptions. They are usually canned without artificial sweetening, and without cooking. Therefore, they still contain much food value.

The following vegetables are to be considered as part of the list of foods that make you:

Turnips, raw	Peas, green	Chard
Asparagus	Artichokes	Celery, raw
Cauliflower	Carrots, raw	Spinach
Cabbage, raw	Okra	Watercress
Beans, string	Radishes	Tomatoes, fresh or canned
Oyster plant	Greens	Cucumbers
Kohlrabi	Parsnips	Squash
Onions, raw	Beets	Pumpkin
Peppers, green	Lettuce	Corn, green

In the above list, please remember that the young, fresh vegetables contain more minerals, more vitamins and more food value than do the old ones. If boiled, baked or fried they are practically worthless, with the exception of tomatoes. It seems impossible to boil, fry, bake or stew the vitamins and minerals out of tomatoes. They are exceptionally good.

FOODS TO EAT SPARINGLY!

The following list consists of acid-forming foods, which when eaten in *very small amounts* are good foods, but they are concentrated foods and should be used very, very sparingly. Many people have enjoyed perfect health by omitting most of them altogether. This list is as follows:

Fish	Beef
Eggs	Rice
Lamb	Rolled oats
Chicken	Cereals
Mutton	Walnuts
Veal	Peanuts
Corn, canned	Bread, whole wheat,
Oysters	bran or rye

When these foods are eaten, be sure they are only 10 percent of the meal; the other 90 percent should consist of fresh raw fruits or fresh raw vegetables. The following is a list of alkaline foods that combine harmoniously with almost any other food, but when eaten in large quantity, they cause congestion and interfere with digestion, and should be eaten sparingly:

Peas, canned	Milk, raw
Molasses	Buttermilk
Olives	Almonds
Lima beans	Beans, canned
Beans, dry (not	Cucumbers
too old)	Cocoanut
Cream, raw	Cheese
Chestnuts	Cottage cheese

The above list unquestionably contains much food value, but as they are very concentrated foods, and the body's requirement for concentrated foods is limited, they should be used sparingly. There is one exception, however. People who do hard manual labor or who exercise vigorously can eat greater quantities of these foods. That is because muscular activity eliminates waste substances that accumulate as a result of rich, concentrated foods.

FOODS THAT BREAK YOU!

People who have had rheumatism, gout, high blood pressure, glaucoma, cataract, diabetes, in fact every conceivable chronic disease, almost invariably eat too many of the following foods that can break you:

Pork	Denatured cereal
Eggs	Tea and coffee
Cheese	Cocoa and chocolate
Salted meats	Beans
Thick soups	Cranberries (sweetened)
White bread	Gooseberries (sweetened)
White sugar	Bananas
Salt in excess	Potatoes, white or sweet
Pastry	Mushrooms
Milk products	Cooked rutabaga
Butter	Cooked turnips
Fat	Cooked cabbage
Sauces	Corned beef
Hot seasoning	Jams, jellies
Cooked vegetables	and preserves

The first item on our list is pork. Remember, a hog is not ready for the market until he is fat enough to bring a good price. Hogs are dirty, filthy animals, eat anything, are very inactive, and the more poisonous they become, the better price they bring. Excessive fat cells are always the more unhealthy cells, because they retain their toxic substances. "Of the fat of the animal thou shalt not eat." The old prophets knew whereof they spoke.

Eggs can be used on a light, therapeutic diet, and certainly egg whites are harmless. But as normally prepared, eggs are very difficult to digest, which results in congestion of the digestive organs. Cheese is practically impossible to digest because of its high fat content. Meat and creamed soups are acid-forming.

White bread is made of the same flour that is used for making paste. No matter what anyone tells you, it is not good food. White sugar is an inorganic substance which clogs the liver, the pancreas and the kidneys. The same is true of salt. You get enough organic salt in fresh fruits and vegetables. The sugar needed by the body is found in fresh fruits. Fruit sugars are easily absorbed and utilized by the cells.

Milk is not a perfect food. It is well-suited to a light therapeutic diet, in many cases, supplying protein and bulk (it is the only liquid that turns into solids in the stomach). It must be used carefully, however, as described in these pages, and not mixed haphazardly with other foods. Otherwise, it becomes a "binding," fatty food that interferes with digestion and causes constipation. Under ordinary circumstances, why be satisfied with a by-product of a cow's digestion when you can have the original whole product in green, leafy vegetables?

Navy or lima beans tend to form mucus and should be omitted from the diet whenever it is possible to obtain fresh vegetables. Denatured breakfast foods do the same thing. Sauces, wines, beer, tarts and pastry are all very pleasing to the taste, but if readers could see some of the rubbish and colon bacteria washed out of the intestines of people who have suffered untold agony as a result of eating these things, it is doubtful they would find them so pleasing. Gooseberries and cranberries are not palatable without sweetening. Add sugar and they ferment. Therapeutically they are juiced, and drunk raw.

Cocoa may taste good, but it clogs the digestive tract. Body tissues cannot use it. The same is true of chocolate. Its high fatty content leads to gall bladder trouble. Mushrooms will not grow except in soil that contains much bacteria. Mushrooms are a living mass of germs, regardless of their low calorie content. Cooked rutabaga and cooked turnips have little if any food value, and the same is true of cooked cabbage and corned beef.

While it is true these vegetables contain useful nutrients, when they are cooked there is practically nothing left except the pulp, which decays and does not digest.

Bananas are really quite good, when tree ripened. The same banana, when picked green, as most bananas are, and allowed to ripen in transit or in storage, becomes a bulky, dead, lifeless starch which cannot do anything but cause congestion, constipation and toxemia.

Raw potatoes have a number of valued medicinal uses. When cooked, however, they are not good food. After a potato has been peeled, sliced, boiled, then mashed, until all the life has been removed, it's not much different from ashes. The best it can do is clog the system. There is no question about this being true. One glance at people who have rheumatism, high blood pressure and other chronic conditions, and you can usually tell that they have been great potato, white bread and meat eaters.

Jams, jellies and preserves form crystals which irritate the bladder, and these small crystals develop into larger crystals which are called stones. White flour, mashed potatoes and sugar also help in the formation of stones. Is it any wonder we have kidney stones, gallstones, stones in the bladder and deposits in the joints? We wouldn't have them if we didn't eat the foods that produce them.

Volumes could be written about why these foods are not good for you. People who eat them grow old very rapidly, many of them become crippled with arthritis, rheumatism and gout. A large number become anemic, others feeble-minded. Glaucoma and cataracts are always found among people who overindulge in the foods that break you.

HOW RAPID CLEANSING FOODS CURE SPECIFIC AILMENTS!

Actually, there is only one disease. And that is the body's attempt to eliminate toxins or poisons. All known diseases are but manifestations of this one disease; only the symptoms vary. Here is a brief description of some of the most common ailments of the stomach and intestines, with instructions as to how each may be permanently and completely remedied.

CONSTIPATION

Constipation is simply a clogging of the small or large intestine. Normally, food is eliminated 10 to 24 hours after it is eaten. Constipation prevents elimination for several days. During this time, much putrefaction and fermentation takes place. Many toxins are generated and absorbed by the bloodstream, and the hard-packed food residue presses against tiny nerve endings in the colon, often producing headaches, fatigue, nausea and a general feeling of discomfort.

The three most important causes of constipation are wrong foods, lack of abdominal exercise and failure to adopt the natural "squat" position when evacuating. Of these, the use of wrong foods deserves the most attention.

Irregularity is most often caused by too many pasty foods which clog up the intestinal tract. In fact, "pastry" is a good name for many white flour products. Its glue-like effect is exactly what you would expect. Mucus-forming foods like milk, cheese and cooked vegetables also have a tendency to cause constipation. The natural way to remedy this condition is to eat a preponderance of raw fruits and vegetables, with these slow-moving foods, to speed up their transit.

Briefly, here's why laxative drugs are no good. They work by irritating the lining of the intestines. To protect itself, the intestines "weep," just as the eye waters when irritated. This liquid creates soft stools and rapid elimination. If frequently used, however, laxatives irritate the intestines to such an extent that an inflamed colon (colitis) or ulcers result. Repeated enemas weaken the colon walls by dilating them with water. Mineral oil dissolves impacted waste, but also washes out vitamins A, D, E and K, causing symptoms ranging from night blindness to frequent colds, skin problems and gall and kidney stones.

The only effective means of completely remedying constipation once and for all, no matter how serious or deep-seated it may be, say drugless doctors, is fruit juice fasting for one or two days, followed by a diet of fresh fruits and vegetables (for details, see Chapter 3).

This will stimulate and cleanse the intestines, and give the intestinal muscles a chance to regain their strength.

Afterwards, white flour products must be avoided, or eaten as sparingly as possible, at the end of the day, for dessert, for example. When you resume eating, there should be plenty of natural fiber in the form of fresh fruits and vegetables. Bran and natural cereals, like shredded wheat are permissible. Whole wheat bread may be eaten in small amounts (high fiber bread is better). Try to move around during the day. At least, stand up and walk a few times. It is the standing up (which is equivalent to bending) that will help you. At home, the squat position can be achieved by placing a small box directly in front of the seat, or by lifting the seat in front with taped blocks of wood, or simply by leaning forward as far as possible.

Rapid cleansing foods that can relieve constipation include:

- High fiber foods, including fresh fruits, nuts, vegetables, seeds, cereals with bran and high fiber bread. One woman says that since eating raw fruit, her lifetime problem of constipation is over, and she has two or three bowel movements a day.

- Papaya can cleanse the intestines and relieve constipation. A woman who tried papaya after everything else failed, including natural bran, says it relieved her constipation completely.

- Sunflower seeds have a laxative effect. Eating a handful, several times a day, can establish regularity in many cases.

- Yellow Dock Tea has brought dramatic relief from constipation. It is an old Chinese remedy. It is available at many health food stores and herbal pharmacies. Even in stubborn cases, results are said to come in a day or so by drinking four to five cups of the hot tea daily, with bulk foods for breakfast. One man says the result was pure magic. Right from the second day on, he had regular bowel movements.

- The simple addition of more water to the diet often relieves constipation in long-standing (20-year) sufferers. A glass of water before orange juice and cereal at breakfast, and at least one more glass of water before bed-time, is usually recommended by doctors.

• Escarole is a powerful laxative that can often relieve intestinal blockage. One method is to drink the water in which escarole has been boiled. It works like magic. Eating some raw, first thing in the morning, can also work amazingly well. Since the vegetable itself is fairly bitter, the pot liquor may be easier to take. One man was so completely constipated he thought he had a growth or polyps or some kind of intestinal blockage. An elderly doctor said frankly, "You don't need any laxatives, or even an operation." He was told to use this method, and from that moment on, he had no pain, no straining and completely natural evacuations.

All of which seems to prove, says one writer, the next time you're in pain, instead of going to your local druggist who'll charge you a fortune and fill you with chemicals, try your local supermarket, where you can get relief for a few cents' worth of fruits, nuts, vegetables or seeds.

HEMORRHOIDS

Constipation often results in hemorrhoids, a bulging of veins in the rectum with congested blood. These are further irritated by laxatives and toxic material from the intestines. Rapid cleansing foods for constipation will go far toward eliminating hemorrhoids, causing them to disappear completely in many cases. Specific foods that have been used to relieve hemorrhoids include cranberries. When all other remedies, including castor oil and vitamin E, fail, cranberries can be counted on for immediate relief. Chop up a handful of cranberries, wrap about a tablespoon or so in a piece of cheesecloth and tuck it in the area. One woman says that within 30 minutes she could feel the pain being drawn out. Repeat at the end of this time. You'll feel great and sleep through the night.

Probably the best local treatment for hemorrhoids, said one doctor, is ice, held to the rectum for two or three minutes at a time. This will contract any enlarged veins, and will also aid the rectal muscles in recovering their normal tone. Afterwards, a glycerine suppository or some cocoa butter should be inserted in the rectum and allowed to remain overnight. This should be continued until the constipation is overcome with a non-constipating diet of rapid cleansing foods.

Vinegar will relieve rectal itching by cleansing the area of germs. Simply saturate a wad of cotton with ordinary vinegar, and apply overnight. It can bring total relief that seems permanent in many cases. (If irritated by scratching there may be a temporary burning sensation.) Wheat germ oil can relieve rectal itching, when all else fails. Wash the area with soap, rinse and dry completely. Then apply wheat germ oil. In severe cases, apply during the day when convenient and repeat the entire procedure at night. Sufferers say soreness and itching vanish.

DIARRHEA

Diarrhea is the body's way of throwing off poisons in a hurry. When you have taken anything into your system which your body cannot tolerate, diarrhea usually results. Drugs which suppress diarrhea force the body to retain these poisons, and while diarrhea can pose an inconvenience, it should not be suppressed by unnatural means. In extreme cases, a natural way to relieve diarrhea quickly is with garlic, which has relieved even the extreme diarrhea of dysentery. Garlic has a powerful cleansing effect on intestinal germs that cause putrefaction. One woman reports: "I had diarrhea for a long time, and was so weak I could hardly move. I felt exhausted and my weight dropped alarmingly. Every time I stopped taking the doctor's prescription, the diarrhea came back, worse than ever. Then I was told to try garlic, by taking a teaspoonful of the diced pieces with milk or honey, two or three times a day. The amazing thing is, my diarrhea ceased almost immediately." Others report the same results.

Ms. P.C. reports: "Diarrhea has plagued me for more than 10 years. The doctors I consulted were unable to help. Their only suggestion was to restrict my diet. Fatty foods gave me the most trouble. The crowning event was a trip to Mexico where I got 'Montezuma's Revenge.' Back home the diarrhea hung on for over a week. I was losing about a half pound a day. Then I talked to a friend who suggested I try acidophilus. I was willing to try anything. In no time at all, after taking acidophilus, I was over the severe diarrhea and even my old problem with fatty foods began to decrease. Within two weeks, I was able to eat without worry."

COLITIS

Laxatives, strong spices, alcoholic beverages, irritating condiments and other factors often give rise to inflammation of the colon or large intestine, known as colitis. The contact of certain rough, coarse or acid foods with the inflamed area often produces much pain and discomfort. Along with this, there are frequently alternating bouts of constipation·and diarrhea, with shreds of mucous streaked with blood in the stools, gas bloating, loss of appetite, foul breath, irritability and weakness. If the colitis is not relieved, an ulcerous sore may develop (ulcerative colitis).

Doctors place practically all colitis patients on a bland diet of soft, mushy foods, including milk, cream, poached eggs, white bread, refined cereals and overcooked, pureed vegetables. This diet does not cure colitis. It relieves pain temporarily, but constipation becomes more severe, with more agony.

There is one remedy and only one remedy for colitis, say drugless doctors. This is fasting (see Chapter 3). Nothing else can produce complete recovery. With this method, the colon is rested, inflammation disappears and tissues heal, they say. Rest and relaxation are advised. Afterward, a wide variety of wholesome, natural foods is suggested. But rapid healing foods alone may help in some cases.

One woman reports: "I am now 33 years old. I was stricken with ulcerative colitis when I was 11 years old. There were many loopholes in what the doctors told me. Pickles and milk, etc., did not bother me . . . and much to their bewilderment, alcoholic beverages caused rectal bleeding . . . I will waste no more time on the past. I switched to whole wheat bread and brown rice and started drinking freshly squeezed orange juice every day. After some time, I realized that I no longer had diarrhea and was apparently absent of the symptoms of my disease. My doctor warned me that, as an ulcerative colitis patient, my chances of developing cancer were 20 percent higher than average. He recommended yearly x-rays to keep a close watch. When my daughter was 2½ years old, I decided it was time to check it . . . I wish I had a tape recorder to record his amazement. The diseased area was completely healed!"

GAS
(Flatulence)

One doctor claimed that 90 percent of his patients complained of gas, and said that this was the symptom they would most like to get rid of. It is fermenting foods which make gas, create noxious poisons and put pressure on many organs. A typical gassy diet would be one in which starches and fruits are eaten together, followed by creamed coffee at meals and in between, or a breakfast consisting of orange juice followed by a dish of oatmeal seasoned with sugar; or gassy foods like beans or cooked cabbage are eaten. A doctor reports this actual case:

> **A woman, 38, was suffering from palpitation of the heart and shortness of breath. Although her weight, 127 lbs., seemed normal for her height, her abdomen measured 48″ when it should have measured about 25″. This was chiefly because her intestines were constantly filled with a large amount of gas. She lost 10 inches in three days, with the following method.**

A fast of grapefruit juice was started, using a glass three times daily, together with a glass of water. After the third day, her abdomen had decreased to 38″. This bloated condition which had been removed was almost entirely gas. The fast was continued for 20 days, during which time the abdomen came down to 24″—exactly half its former size. She was then put upon the following diet:

Breakfast—Whites of 3 eggs.
　　　　　3 or 4 slices of thin, brown toast.
　　　　　Choice of stewed fruit, without sugar.
Lunch—　Glass of orange juice, with a glass of water.
Dinner—　One of the following: lean beef, chicken, turkey, rabbit or lean fish.
　　　　　2 non-starch vegetables.
　　　　　Raw celery.

There was no further bloated appearance from gas pressure. Toning up exercises were used, until the abdomen was again of a normal contour. Constipation, which had existed for many years, was entirely overcome, and a partial obstruction of the lower bowels was removed, which was responsible for a good deal of gas accumulation. She is still in perfect health after many years.

ULCERS

An ulcer is a crater-like sore in the wall of the stomach or intestine. The gastric juice of the ulcer patient is always too acid, and helps produce the sore. In fact, this acid condition pervades the entire body. It is due largely to overeating acid-forming foods, such as cereals, bread, meat, cheese, eggs, coffee. Medical doctors are not sure of what causes ulcers, but they treat it with the Sippy diet, which consists of taking milk and cream every two hours, with bland foods and alkaline powders. These bland foods are acid-forming (you must realize that foods with an acid taste are neutralized in the body, and are called alkaline; and foods with a bland taste become mixed with acids in the system, and are said to be acid-forming).

Neither bland foods nor alkaline powders will cure a stomach ulcer, as I can tell you from personal experience. Relief is temporary, and symptoms return with great force. Most patients agree. Some resort to surgery. The surgeon removes the ulcer or makes a new opening which drains the acids away from the original spot. After temporary relief, the ulcer patient returns to his old way of eating and develops a new ulcer.

Drugless doctors say that one way to cure an ulcer is to fast, which gives the affected area an opportunity to heal. The treatment is similar to that used in treating colitis. After the fast a highly alkaline fruit and vegetable diet is used, along with exercise and sunbathing. With this method, say drugless doctors, recovery may be expected in all except the most severe cases, and even they experience great improvement.

Rapid healing or rapid cleansing foods are also used by drugless doctors to create an effect similar to fasting, without the inconvenience of going without food. These foods help the body cleanse itself, because they are so easy to digest. They give the body a rest, a chance to heal. Some of them contain important healing factors. For example, cabbage contains the anti-ulcer vitamin U, plus chlorine and sulfur which help cleanse the mucous membranes of the stomach. This, say researchers, is only possible if eaten raw or its fresh juice drunk. This treatment is now recognized by many doctors.

A man with two stomach ulcers tried it. He started with five glasses of raw cabbage juice the first day and almost at once, there was no pain. He tapered off to three glasses daily after a week. Both ulcers were healed when he had his check-up x-rays two months later. A man with an acute peptic ulcer—awaiting surgery—was told by his doctor to drink a quart of fresh cabbage juice (four glasses) daily, for immediate relief. In a few days, he felt so good surgery was avoided.

Comfrey, a common tea, possesses extraordinary healing powers due to a substance in it called allantoin. It can heal bleeding ulcers. In one miraculous case, a man suffering pain after food, vomiting of blood and other ulcer symptoms, with no relief from medicines, finally agreed to an operation. He nearly died on the operating table, and surgery had to be stopped (the ulcer remaining). He was then treated with allantoin in a comfrey infusion (tea) and a purely milk diet, and was completely free of ulcers in a month. In another case, a woman with a bleeding ulcer tried it. All she did was sip strong comfrey tea until she felt well. In a matter of days, she was completely healed, without medicines.

Honey has cured many hopeless cases of gastric and intestinal ulcers, without operations, says a medical doctor, adding that the news has not yet reached 99% of the medical profession and those who do know it are afraid to say so for fear of being laughed at. Father Kneipp, the great naturalist, always claimed that small ulcers are healed by honey. A man who suffered for years from an ulcerated stomach, in and out of hospitals and in much pain, noticed that after eating honey he felt much better, kept eating it and never had any relapse.

Okra heals ulcers, due to its thick, gooey nature when cooked or used in soup. This mucilaginous liquid helps neutralize hydrochloric acid. It is also good for colitis (inflammation of the colon), relieving the attacks of constipation and diarrhea. Of 17 persons with ulcer of the stomach or the first part of the intestines who were given powdered okra as the only form of treatment, 14 received immediate relief. It not only eased the discomfort, but caused the stomach to empty more promptly.

Alfalfa tea has been used to heal ulcers. The treatment consists of 1 tablespoon of powdered alfalfa in a glass of water, once a day; 1 teaspoon of olive oil before meals; and no fried foods, bread or alcohol. One woman with stomach pains caused by an ulcer—threatened with an operation—says this method gave her immediate relief, and in a few weeks her stomach ulcer had completely healed, as confirmed by x-rays.

Among various home remedies reported by men and women in all walks of life, goat milk was used by an ulcer sufferer who'd been told by 15 doctors that his case was "incurable." His ulcers completely disappeared, as confirmed by x-rays. Celery has been used to relieve heartburn and indigestion. One woman with diverticulitis, suffering upset stomach and acid rising into her throat, discovered that one large radish acts like magic, instantly quieting all symptoms of indigestion.

Rapid healing foods have also been used as follows:

- Papaya can cleanse the stomach and intestines of decayed, fetid or putrefying protein wastes that have been only partially digested, with a powerful digestive enzyme called papain. An invaluable aid for feeble digestion, it helps clear up gas, heartburn and diarrhea, helps digest meat, eggs and protein, and is actually used as a meat tenderizer.

- Cucumbers contain an enzyme called erepsin which aids in digestion of proteins. Their actual protein digestion power is comparable to that of papaya.

- Pineapple contains bromelain, a powerful enzyme good for digesting meat. It helps relieve indigestion and upset stomach. Persimmons soothe stomach and intestinal ulcers. Nectarines aid digestion and relieve gas, as do endives and tomatoes. The juice of raw carrots, tomatoes, celery and potatoes has been used to relieve ulcers. Other foods that relieve ulcers include cocoanut milk, dates and eggplant.

Drinking great quantities of water and fruit juices without sugar for one day will not only cleanse the intestinal tract, but also tends to cleanse all the cells of the body. If it is continued a second day, much more waste substance and toxic material is eliminated. Your food, in many cases, is responsible for the way you feel. Live principally on the foods that make you, and eliminate from the diet the foods that break you, and you will cleanse and strengthen all of your organs of digestion and elimination.

RAPID HEALING FOODS FOR STOMACH AND INTESTINES!

Here is a complete breakdown of foods that have been used to relieve stomach and intestinal problems:

Constipation

artichokes,
   Jerusalem
avocado
bamboo shoots
beet greens
beet juice (red)
blackberries
blueberries
bran
bread, high fiber
broccoli
Brussels sprouts
cabbage, raw, juice
cantaloupe
carrots, raw, juice
cauliflower
celery, raw, juice
chard
cherries
cocoanuts
collards
corn
cranberries
cucumber juice,
   raw
dandelion tea
eggplant
elderberry
escarole
figs
garlic
grapes
lettuce
loquat
millet
mustard greens
nettle tea

olives
onions
papaya
pears
pepper, green
persimmon
pineapple
plum
prunes
pumpkin seeds
quince
radishes
raisins
raspberries
rhubarb
rutabaga
sauerkraut
sesame seeds
squash, summer
strawberries
sunflower seeds
tomato
walnuts
water
water chestnuts
Yellow Dock tea

Colitis

bananas
bread, whole wheat
carrots
dates
eggplant
okra
parsnips
pears
persimmon

potato, sweet
rice, brown
tapioca

Cramps

artichokes,
   Jerusalem
cantaloupe
cherries
cocoanuts
garlic
olives
plum
rutabaga
water chestnut

Diarrhea

bananas
blueberries
garlic
papaya
potato, sweet
rice, brown

Dysentery

beet greens
blackberries
blueberries
cocoanut milk
garlic

Gas

artichoke,
   Jerusalem

cantaloupe
cocoanuts
endives
nectarines
olives
papaya
plum
rutabaga
tomato
water chestnuts

Heartburn
(see Ulcers)

Hemorrhoids

bananas
cranberries
   (external)

persimmon
potato, sweet
prunes

Ulcers

alfalfa tea
banana
cabbage juice, raw
carrot juice, raw
celery
cocoanut milk
comfrey tea
dates
eggplant
honey
milk

okra
parsnips
persimmon
pineapple
potato, sweet
radish
rice, brown
tapioca

Worms

garlic
pineapple
pumpkin seeds
rutabagas
sesame seeds
water chestnuts

3

Rapid Healing Foods
to Cleanse
Your System!

Astonishing as it may seem, fasting is actually rapid healing, rapid cleansing food for the body. During a fast, excess waste, sludge and debris in the body—actually the protein in them—become food for the body and this rubbish is burned up and eliminated.

A cleansing diet of certain liquid and natural foods will help rid your body of accumulated rubbish, say many experts—and this is what is meant by fasting, as practiced today in many great European health spas. It is a far cry from starvation, and has miraculously cured almost every known ailment!

Many times, a single food seems specific for certain ailments, and that food is used, for a short time, on a mono-diet which gives your delicate glands and organs both a cleansing and a much-needed rest from work which has been going on day and night for many years. After a cleansing diet, normal hunger soon returns for wholesome bulk foods, replacing your cravings for the greasy, starchy, sweet and fast food items that brought on your distress in the first place.

HOW POISONS ARE ELIMINATED!

During a cleansing diet, a process called autolysis takes place. Autolysis is the self-loosening and elimination of unwanted waste. Special enzymes are produced in the body which have the power to dissolve hardened infusions, encrustations and crystallized deposits.

These digestive enzymes are carried by the blood to each and every cell of the body, where they soon begin a cleansing action. Even cholesterol deposits within the blood vessels are melted and carried away. Waste deposits in all other parts of the body are liquefied, carried off and eliminated.

As one expert states: "First (during a cleansing diet), after the first three days . . . the body will decompose and burn only those substances and tissues which are diseased, damaged or of lesser importance . . . such as all morbid accumulations, tumors, abscesses, damaged tissues, fat deposits, etc . . . Second . . . masses of accumulated metabolic wastes and toxins are quickly expelled . . . (Lastly) the nervous system is regenerated, mental powers improved, glandular chemistry and secretions are normalized."[1] Proof that wastes are being eliminated is that during the first few days, you may experience bad breath, darker urine (concentration of toxins in the urine is 10 times higher than normal), frequent bowel movements, perspiration and perhaps some mucus or phlegm.[2] But after a day or so, the breath becomes sweet, the tongue clear, the body cleansed and rejuvenated.

EASY CLEANSING DIETS
TO HEAL AND REVITALIZE
YOUR VITAL ORGANS!

Cleansing diets are really very simple. They range from the simplest use of water, and nothing else, for 24 hours, to a fruit

---

[1]*Health Secrets from Europe*, by Paavo Airola, N.D. (Parker Publishing Company, Inc., West Nyack, N.Y.), 1970.

[2]Op. cit.

juice fast for the same length of time. Another method is to eat nothing but fresh fruits for a day or so. On the first day of such a fast the cells will let loose some of their poison. On the second day more poison will be eliminated. This is thrown into the intestinal tract and is filtered out by the kidneys and bowels. Here is a suggested one-day cleansing diet that permits you to eat with pleasure and satisfaction:[3]

BEFORE BREAKFAST. Take half a glass of raw potato juice diluted with room temperature water. (Grate potatoes and strain out the juice.)

BREAKFAST . . . . Bowl of whole wheat that has been soaked in water for two or three days. Make more palatable with a good vegetable stock. Whole grain bread with soya butter and sprinkled with wheat germ flakes. To improve bowel function, add psyllium or freshly ground linseeds to the wheat.

LUNCHEON. . . . . A good, strong vegetable soup with about one glass (average 8 oz.) of raw and freshly squeezed cabbage juice added, after the soup has been taken off the fire. Now a dish of steamed brown (unpolished) rice, bowl of millet, steamed seasonal vegetables that cannot be eaten raw and a portion of raw fresh vegetables. For salad dressing, use lemon juice mixed with apple cider vinegar. If you are troubled with nervous conditions, beat a raw egg until fluffy and add to a glass of freshly squeezed grapefruit juice.

---

[3]*The Natural Way to Health Through Controlled Fasting*, by Carlson Wade (Parker Publishing Company, Inc., West Nyack, N.Y.), 1968.

DINNER .... This may be similar to your breakfast. You can vary the whole wheat dish by taking oat porridge—or put raw, soaked oats through a blender and eat with a spoon.

This one-day cleansing diet menu permits you to eat, but is carefully composed of easily digested foods that leave little waste residue. You can fast and enjoy food at the same time! A simpler method is not to go on any specific diet, but just cut out meat, eliminate all highly seasoned gravy, rich cake and sugary preserves.[4]

A DO-IT-YOURSELF PROGRAM!

Most recognized authorities state that, while a liquid or juice diet is not dangerous and could be undertaken at home, for safety's sake it is best to do so under a doctor's supervision. In Scandinavia, cleansing diets are a national sport. These short diets are considered to be an effective way to cleanse the body of wastes, avoid illness and build resistance to disease. In his book, *Health Secrets from Europe*, Paavo Airola gives a short description of a juice diet.

First, it is advisable to prepare yourself by a short cleansing diet. "For two or three days, eat only raw fruits and vegetables, alternating one meal made up of any available fruits with a meal of vegetables.

"On the day before the main diet, take a dose of castor oil in the early afternoon to clean the bowels, and do not eat any dinner. Before going to bed take a double enema. First, take one pint of plain water at body temperature, and let it out. Then repeat with a full quart. If you can make camomile tea and mix it with water, so much the better. Camomile can be obtained at drugstores or health food stores. Enemas during fasting are very important. They help the body in the elimination of toxins and waste matter from the colon and lower bowels—and you will be amazed at the amount of waste coming out with the enema even after two or three weeks of fasting!

---

[4]Op. cit.

"The next day, and each following day (of the main cleansing diet) you follow this program:

Upon Arising: Cup of herb tea—lukewarm, not hot. Health food stores usually have a large assortment of herb teas. Use the instructions on the package for preparing them. Peppermint, camomile, rose hips and red clover are some of the teas which can be used.

9 to 10 a.m.: Glass of freshly squeezed fruit juice: orange, apple, grape, pear, etc . . . Practically any fruit juice can be used, but try to use those which are specifically beneficial for your condition [see examples in coming chapters]. Juice should be diluted half-and-half with water. NOTE! Avoid commercially bottled, canned or frozen juices.

1:00 p.m.: Glass of freshly made vegetable juice: carrot, celery, tomato, etc., or a mixture of several vegetable juices. Dilute with water. Or a cup of vegetable broth.

4:00 p.m.: Cup of herb tea.

7:00 p.m.: Glass of freshly made vegetable or fruit juice, diluted with water.

9:00 p.m.: Enema, preferably camomile.

"Drink plain lukewarm water when thirsty. The total juice volume during 24 hours should be between 1½ pints and 1½ quarts. Never mix fresh juices with vegetable broth, only with pure water.

"This is all. You may show these instructions to your own doctor and ask him to supervise your fasting and examine your condition as your fasting progresses. If you are not able to obtain expert advice, and if you, yourself, are not sufficiently convinced of the safety and efficiency of this healing measure, I would not advise you to fast longer than one week to 10 days at a time."

COMPLETING A
CLEANSING DIET!

Dr. Airola stresses that this is the most important part of a cleansing diet. Its beneficial effects would be totally undone if ended incorrectly. The main rules to follow, he says, are:

- Do not overeat!
- Chew food extremely well and eat slowly!
- Take several days of gradual transition to the normal diet!

On the first day, he suggests, eat one whole apple or other sweet fruit and a little bowl of fresh vegetable soup or puree, unsalted and unspiced, in addition to the usual juice and broth menu. On the second day, add some mashed potatoes and a glass of yogurt or homemade soured milk. On the third day, increase the portions a little and add a small plate of fresh raw vegetable salad, some cooked rice and a little portion of homemade cottage cheese. On the fourth day, you can start to eat normally, but do not overeat, he stresses.

MORE ADVICE ...

Should you discontinue work, or stay in bed, during a cleansing diet? Not at all, says Dr. Airola: "It is advisable to continue with your usual activities, but perhaps avoid too strenuous physical and mental work. Daily walks, even long ones for an hour or more, twice a day, are recommended ... Take a bath two or three times a week, but avoid water too cold or too hot."

Your mental attitude is extremely important, says Dr. Airola: "Do not listen to terrified relatives and friends who will warn you that you will pass out at any moment ... nobody has ever died as a result of a few weeks of intentional fasting. Have confidence in what you are doing. Remember, you are not the first to try it—millions of people have done it successfully before you. Even animals fast instinctively when they are sick. But if you do not have complete faith in fasting and are not absolutely convinced of its safety, you should not undertake it at all, at least not on your own." However, if you do, he adds, "I know you will be surprised at the results."

MANY AILMENTS VANISH!

An astonishing number of ailments have been relieved, and seemingly hopeless cases cured, by the cleansing diet. Stomach and intestinal disorders, ulcers, colitis, chronic constipation, liver and gall bladder problems, kidney, bladder and urinary problems, diabetes, heart, vein and artery problems, high blood pressure, anemia, edema, leg ulcers, arthritic and rheumatic complaints, lung problems, respiratory ailments, skin disorders, even cases of extreme overweight, have all responded well to a cleansing diet.

> **The benefits of rapid healing, rapid cleansing foods are well known. According to the British Ministry of Health, for example: "Juices are valuable to relief of hypertension, cardiovascular and kidney diseases and obesity. Good results have also been obtained in rheumatism, degenerative and toxic states. Juices have an all-around protective action. Good results can be obtained when large amounts up to one quart daily are taken in treatment of peptic ulceration, also in treatment of chronic diarrhea, colitis and toxemia of gastro and intestinal origin."**

Doctors have noted the general well-being of sufferers who have been on a cleansing diet, and many a doctor advises it as the speediest way to rid the body of certain toxins and impurities or to overcome a cold or the flu. A cleansing diet establishes a good elimination, and ulcers, colitis and other digestive ailments often disappear. It will also give your pancreas a rest. The heart is relieved of the vigorous pumping required to digest heavy meals. Those who follow a cleansing diet acquire a much clearer skin, and acne, psoriasis and recurrent skin infections may be relieved (although during the first few days there may be skin eruptions as poisons are thrown off). Warm baths during a cleansing diet help eliminate noxious poisons from the body.

One doctor suggests going on a cleansing raw fruit diet at the first sign of a cold—a diet consisting entirely of fruits or fruit juices—for two days. You may have all the fruit or fruit juices you wish, any variety. A person on a cleansing diet, he says, never catches a cold, and if you have one, it will rapidly clear up during a fruit diet. During a cleansing diet consisting of fruits and water, according to one medical authority, germs are burned up or oxidized and eliminated and great quantities of mucus will be eliminated from the lungs. A cleansing diet can be used any time, any place, at home or away, by simply eating only fresh raw fruits and juices at the first sign of a cold or virus infection. You will then dissolve these germs, burn them up and eliminate them, he says.

SWELLINGS, FLUID, GROWTHS
DISAPPEAR!

Poisons from decomposed food which are not expelled from the intestines are often reabsorbed by the blood and carried elsewhere. Some of these poisons accumulate to form boils, stones, pimples and various other types of growths. By means of a cleansing diet, many people have gotten rid of body growths. Non-cancerous tumors can be disintegrated by a cleansing diet. Body fat and bumps (fatty tumors) often disappear. Years ago, Bernarr Macfadden noted—

"My experience of (cleansing diets) has shown me beyond all possible doubt that a foreign growth of practically any kind can be absorbed into the body's circulation by simply compelling the body to use unnecessary elements contained within it for food. When a foreign growth has become hardened, sometimes (a cleansing diet) will not accomplish the result, but where they are soft, the (cleansing diet) will usually cause them to be absorbed."

During a cleansing diet, dropsical swellings, edematous swellings and deposits are absorbed, says Carlson Wade. A cleansing diet will cause a more rapid absorption of dropsical fluid which has accumulated in the tissues than any other known measure, he says. A skin lesion (sore) may cease growing, its size eventually reduced or completely absorbed during a cleansing diet, he adds.[5]

NATURE'S SUPREME HEALING AGENT!

The cleansing diet is perhaps the greatest health discovery of the last century. It is really the most rapid and effective means of healing many diseases. It is often called "the fast way to health" and is recommended for those who desire to become well in the shortest possible time, say drugless doctors. Orthodox medical doctors consider fasting too fantastic to be given any serious consideration. It is placed on their list of "fads." But for non-medical doctors, it has become the foundation

---

[5]*Ibid.*

of drugless healing. It remains nature's greatest healing force and the only hope many sick people may have.

> Actual cell tissue rejuvenation takes place during a cleansing diet, and this has been proven in tests at the University of Chicago. Many abnormal growths are removed on a cleansing diet, and this disintegration of growths has been noted again and again. Tumors as large as a goose egg have disappeared on diets of a few weeks' duration. Small growths the size of a pea usually disappear after three or four days. This has been observed in thousands of cases in Europe and America.

Dr. Herbert M. Shelton, of San Antonio, Texas, treated over 20,000 patients with cleansing diets. The people who came to him were largely those who had tried everything else—medicine, surgery, chiropractic—all to no avail. For them, the cleansing diet was a last resort. Their ailments included heart disease, ulcers, colitis, asthma, sinusitis, tumors and arthritis. Dr. Shelton reported that 95 percent of these patients were relieved or cured.

The noted writer, Upton Sinclair, once took a survey of 117 people who used cleansing diets for relief of health problems. These people reported the following diseases relieved or cured:

Nervousness	27
Constipation	14
Colds	8
Catarrh	6
Neurasthenia	6
Rheumatism	5
Bronchial trouble	5
Headaches	5
Liver trouble	5
General debility	5
Tuberculosis	4
Anemia	3
Poor circulation	3
Appendicitis	3
Uric acid excess	2
Syphilis	1
Scrofula	1
Cancer	1
Gas poisoning	1
Insomnia	1

Grippe 1
Valvular disease of the heart......................... 1
Pleurisy... 1
Epilepsy 1
Asthma 1
Sciatica 1
Locomotor ataxia 1
Blood poisoning...................................... 1
Chills and fever..................................... 1
Ulcerated leg.. 1

Only 14 percent were not helped. They failed to follow instructions or went back to their old eating habits.

Reportedly, many so-called incurable diseases that baffle scientists readily yield to a cleansing diet. In leper colonies under strict medical supervision recoveries are extremely rare. But in as little as 21 days on a cleansing diet, leprosy has been completely remedied. One writer reports: "Heart disease and cancer, two of the most common degenerative diseases for which medical science can do little or nothing, often yield to fasting if not allowed to become too far advanced. Leukemia and Bright's disease, long considered incurable, respond favorably to fasting." Even gonorrhea has been cured!

One medical doctor states that he has seen complete cures, in a short time, with a cleansing diet, for such diseases as chronic eczema, uticaria, varicose ulcers, gastric and duodenal ulcers, asthma, arthritis, colitis, amebic dynsentery, endocarditis, sinusitis, bronchitis, neuritis, Bright's disease, tic douloureux, fistula, psoriasis, all kinds of digestive disorders, gallstones, kidney stones, bladder stones, glaucoma, breast lumps, migraine, acidosis, epilepsy, Parkinson's disease (shaking palsy), Renaud's disease and much more. He says it's the closest thing to a cure-all known to mankind!

Another doctor reports that hearing has been regained in ears that were deaf for years, eyeglasses have been discarded, facial lines vanished, blood pressure reduced, heart action improved, prostate glands normalized, in case after case with a cleansing diet. It can bring about a virtual rebirth, he emphasizes! And for the reducer, weight-loss of 4 to 6 pounds a day is possible (2½ pounds average), and a loss of 20 pounds in a week is not at all difficult in a great many cases, he says!

HOW SAFE IS IT?

In his book, *Health Secrets from Europe*, Dr. Paavo Airola states that, although the cleansing diet is without doubt one of the safest healing agents known to medicine, in the minds of the uninitiated and uninformed it is often associated with fear of doing harm to the body. Nobody ever died as a result of a cleansing diet, he points out. Naturally, if you are suffering from a serious condition such as cancer, tuberculosis, diabetes, or cardiovascular disorders, you should be at all times under a doctor's supervision, he adds, but otherwise a cleansing diet—particularly a juice diet—can be safely undertaken by anyone. Dr. Airola says that he, himself, has used this method countless times and can testify that it not only works, but is indeed one of the safest healing methods there is.

4

Rapid Healing Foods for Heart, Veins and Arteries!

Poisonous waste shows up in heart disorders in the form of degeneration of the heart muscle, hardening of the coronary arteries, irregular heartbeat, overgrowth of the heart tissue, dilatation or enlargement of heart and vessels. All of these are effects stemming from saturation or choking of the tissues with excessive waste products. Cholesterol, a gooey sludge derived from fat, eggs and meat, seems to make up the greatest amount of these choking materials. Uric acid and various forms of calcium have also been identified in the mass of waste products.

In angina pectoris or coronary occlusion, the amount of clogging debris has reached such critical proportions that circulation is almost completely blocked. One naturopathic doctor who made a close study of several hundred cases of heart ailments, including his own, claims that complete food abstinence or the water diet is the quickest way to help the heart back to normal.

After the sixth or seventh day, he says, an amazing change

takes place. The feeling of fullness or congestion becomes less noticeable. Pains that have spread into the left upper arm disappear. Irregular beatings tend to become normalized. The heart grows stronger every hour as the load it has been carrying is lessened, he says. Naturally, no one with heart trouble should ever undertake such a fast without medical supervision, but...

AMAZING RECOVERIES CLAIMED!

This researcher states that in his own case, he was suffering from a persistent heart condition. The slightest physical exertion resulted in sharp, penetrating pains in the heart, due to a coronary occlusion. A naturopathic doctor advised a cleansing diet, as described above. In five days, he says, he lost all pain in the upper chest. Not only his heart, but every fiber of his body felt rejuvenated. This happened 25 years ago, he says, and ever since that time his heart has been normal. On this subject, Hereward Carrington, Ph.D., author of *Vitality, Fasting and Nutrition*, says:

> **"That the heart is invariably strengthened and invigorated by fasting is true beyond a doubt. I take the stand that fasting is the greatest of all strengtheners of weak hearts—being, in fact, its only rational physiological care."**

The foremost authority on cleansing diets, Dr. Herbert Shelton has stated that in the hundreds of cases of heart disease he has treated with this method, almost all developed stronger and better hearts. Many of them, even so-called *incurable* ones, have become entirely normal, he says. Rapid hearts have slowed down, abnormally slow hearts have speeded up, weak hearts have greatly improved in vigor, hearts that were irregular have become regular—all due to the rest that fasting brings from the furious beating of the heart during heavy meals, a decrease of burdensome pounds, elimination of excess fluids and high blood pressure and a seemingly instantaneous improvement in kidney function.

One patient, a 24-year-old man had a clinical diagnosis of mitral stenosis. He was in grave condition, with failure largely on the right side of his heart. His heart and liver were greatly enlarged. The usual medications gave no relief. Then he was given a fast for seven days. In three days he was greatly improved. His liver reduced in size at the rate of two finger-breadths a day for a week. Kidney function greatly improved. Excess fluid vanished in a week.

VALVULAR TROUBLES

Many persons, unaware of any heart defect, often suffer general weakness, shortness of breath and poor circulation, without realizing that these may be caused by heart valve defects. In some cases the valves have become narrowed or hardened, so that they cannot close completely. In other cases, inflammation of the lining of the heart exists. Drugless doctors cite the following as the principal causes of heart valve trouble:

1. Birth defects.
2. Streptococcus infections, such as those that result in inflammation of the lining of the heart and rheumatic fever.
3. Any enlargement which interferes with the free circulation of blood and causes undue strain upon the heart.
4. Overeating of all kinds of food, and drinking too much fluid, improper food combinations and principally the use of too much starch and sugar.

Reportedly, fasting has been used successfully in hundreds of cases for relief of symptoms, one drugless doctor going so far as to say: "Every case will be benefited, and I have records of many hopeless patients who were restored to perfect health through this method." In order to give the heart a rest, said this doctor, it is advisable to fast from all food except the juice of acid fruit for a few days, after which the patient should use a diet free from all gas-forming food, and eliminate all starch and sugar. Reduce fluid intake, especially when dropsy is present, he said, adding that weight must be kept down to avoid needless strain upon the heart. Early dinners for complete digestion before sleep, and keeping the feet warm at night to aid circulation, are recommended.

This doctor reported the following case: "A young woman, 35, had been troubled with cold hands and feet for years, and could not go bathing without having her lips and fingernails turn blue. She felt very weak most of the time, and was unable to do any regular work. She'd been turned down for life insurance because of valvular leakage of the heart. I found she had a prolapsed (sagging) stomach and intestines, and that she was troubled with a good deal of stomach and intestinal gas. I felt this gas pressure was responsible for her heart trouble, and that if she followed my diet the gas would be removed.

"She accordingly started on a fruit-juice fast, drinking nothing but water, in each glass of which she squeezed a few drops of lemon juice. No other food or liquid of any kind was taken for 15 days. At the end of that time the blood pressure, which had been 110 millimeters systolic, rose to 115 millimeters, and she felt better in every way. She was then put on a milk diet, using 3 quarts daily of pure Holstein milk, taken in the raw, unpasteurized state, at the rate of one glass every hour during the day until 3 quarts had been taken. Before each glass of milk the patient took a teaspoonful of lemon juice, which aids in the digestion of milk. This diet was continued for 30 days, and at the end of that time she was given a diet of the following:

Breakfast—2 coddled eggs.
　　　　　3 slices of brown, thin toast.
　　　　　Dish of stewed fruit, selected from the following list: prunes, raisins, figs, apricots, baked or stewed apple.

Lunch—　One quart of milk taken one glass at a time every 15 minutes until the four 8-ounce glasses in the quart are taken. At this lunch of milk she also used a quarter of a pound of raisins.

Dinner—　Choice of one of the following protein foods: chicken, turkey, rabbit, fish.

　　　　　One of the following cooked non-starchy vegetables:

Summer squash	Celery
Small green string beans	Swiss chard
Spinach	Asparagus
Eggplant	Oyster plant
Beet tops	Turnip tops
Kale	Mustard greens
Cucumbers	Chayotes
French artichokes	Parsley
Zucchini	Lettuce

Choice of one of the following raw or salad vegetables:

Watercress	Parsley
Asparagus	Lettuce
Cucumbers	Endive
Spinach	Tomatoes
Celery	

"After several weeks of this diet, combined with osteopathic treatment and massage, also the proper electro-therapy treatment, she was restored to normal, and I could not discover any sign of the valvular trouble in the heart. She has since passed an examination in one of the largest insurance companies and is working in their office, remaining in perfect health."

FATTY HEART

We are all familiar with the headline seen so often in the morning paper: "Mr. Prominent Citizen, apparently in the best of health, sat down to read the evening paper after a hearty dinner, and was found dead in his chair." After this, a list of his virtues follows, and never a word about the cause of death, which was in all probability a so-called "fatty heart." The headline should have read:

"Mr. Over-Fed stuffed himself to death last night, and cheated himself, his family and his community of what might have been a useful citizen."

A fatty heart comes from overindulging and lack of physical exercise. This brings on the typical case of fatty enlargement of the heart, which will result in sudden death as soon as the pressure of fat and gases against the heart becomes too great. Sometimes there is warning in advance by such symptoms as shortness of breath, palpitation upon exertion and discomfort when lying on the left side; but often these are not noticed soon enough. The cure is simple and depends almost entirely upon reducing the weight.

A man of 40, weighing 206 lbs, was unable to sleep at night because of the discomfort he experienced when lying down. The palpitations of his heart were very noticeable. Examination revealed an enlarged, fatty heart. He was put on the following simple diet: one or two sliced tomatoes three times daily, taken in place of other meals. One glass of water was allowed with each meal of tomatoes, and no other food of any kind was taken. This diet was continued for exactly a month, during which time he lost 36 pounds. A re-examination of his heart by x-rays showed it had been reduced at least 2 inches in diameter. His breathing was perfectly normal, and there was no sign of any palpitation. He has remained at about 170 lbs., normal for a man his height.

TACHYCARDIA, RAPID HEART

"The cause of this condition," said one drugless doctor, "is to be found in valvular leakage of the heart, which makes the extra heart beats necessary in order to disseminate the blood properly through the tissues as in an enlargement of some organ of the body such as the thyroid, or the growth of a tumor. Such enlargements are caused by the collection of waste material in the organ, which blocks the free circulation of blood through the part, resulting in an engorgement of blood and a consequent heavy, rapid pulse beat, which is essential in order to force enough blood through the body in spite of this resistance. The cure depends upon the absorption of the deposits, which is best accomplished through ... fasting methods. The following case will show how quickly the heart beat may be reduced to normal.

"A young woman, 25, had a racing pulse of 120. Examination revealed an enlarged thyroid and a slight valvular leakage of the heart—which would account for the rapid pulse. The patient was put on a fast, taking a glass of grapefruit juice three times daily together with a glass of water. This was continued for three weeks, during which time the pulse gradually reduced until at the end of the third week it had reached the normal, which is about 72 beats per minute. The enlargement of the thyroid entirely disappeared, and no signs of valvular heart trouble could be detected. She then resumed a well-balanced diet, and has since passed a rigid test for insurance with flying colors."

HIGH BLOOD PRESSURE

High blood pressure has many causes, but drugless doctors stress a build-up of waste products in the circulatory system as the main cause. It is important to reduce high blood pressure, because it almost invariably leads to trouble in the form of a stroke, clot, hemorrhage, kidney failure, heart failure or sudden death if not controlled. Drugs do exactly this. By dilating or widening the arteries, they lower blood pressure, but do not cure the condition. They must be taken religiously.

Fasting speedily lowers blood pressure, improves circulation and brings not just temporary but permanent relief, in many cases, say drugless doctors. "I have never had a case under my observation," says one such doctor, "where the pressure was not reduced to normal by this method." You can expect to reap the benefits which thousands have received, he says.

Whatever the cause, says this doctor, it may be cured with rapid healing foods, starting with a fruit juice fast: "The thickening of the walls (of the arteries) or deposits on the walls is caused in every case by a toxic state of the blood, which is produced by dietetic errors. In every case the patient has been a heavy starch and sugar eater, and after the fast, when the pressure is reduced to normal, the permanency of the cure depends entirely upon the regulation of the use of carbohydrates, and often upon their elimination.

"I have made elaborate tests to prove this theory, having patients use carbohydrates one day and not the next, and I have been able to tell the day the carbohydrates were used, by blood pressure alone. It is advisable to diminish the intake of liquids if no kidney disease exists, as this will reduce the volume of blood and relieve some of the arterial tension. The bowels must be kept open by enemas if necessary, and the skin encouraged to eliminate properly by sponge or shower baths." He reports the following cases—

"A 67-year-old man had systolic blood pressure of 265 mm. The pressure in his head was so high that he had been unable to lie down for over two weeks, and what little sleep he was able to get was taken sitting in a Morris chair. The blood pressure had affected his brain, so that the power of speech was impaired, and he could not make himself understood.

"The patient was immediately put on an orange juice fast, using the juice of an orange every two hours with a glass of water each time, and taking one enema and one sponge bath each day.

Within a month, his blood pressure was reduced to 125 mm systolic pressure. Then the patient was put on the following diet:

Breakfast—2 eggs.
   3 pieces thin, dry, brown toast.
   Dish of stewed prunes or figs.
Lunch— Choice of a mixture of the following nonstarchy salad vegetables: Swiss chard, green string beans, spinach, asparagus, oyster plant, beet tops, turnip tops, kale, celery, lettuce, cucumber, parsley, carrots, turnips, parsnips, beets.
Dinner— Choice of one of the following: lean beef, chicken, fish, rabbit.
   Choice of 2 cooked nonstarchy vegetables from the following class: spinach, asparagus, summer squash, string beans, lettuce, celery, cucumber.
   Choice of one or more of the following salad vegetables: lettuce, celery, cucumber, tomatoes.
   No dessert.

"A diet similar to this has been continued for the past eight and one-half years without an increase in blood pressure (which is always between 125 and 130 mm). I wish you would especially note in this case that the cure was permanent, and the patient has remained in good health ever since.

"A married woman, 42, suffered from pains in the head, as though an iron band were clamped tightly around the skull. She had profuse menstruation, which continued most of the month with very few intervals in which it stopped entirely. Systolic blood pressure was 228 mm. I explained to her that I believed high blood pressure was producing the excessive bleeding (actually, to relieve still higher pressure and avoid rupture of a blood vessel in the brain). A fast was started on a glass of grapefruit juice taken three times daily, with a glass of water. The usual enemas and sponge baths were taken, and the blood pressure reduced to 125 mm systolic in four days. After several more days, she resumed a well-balanced diet, using a selection similar to the one just given.

"Her blood pressure has remained normal for about a year and a half. Menstruation has entirely ceased, and she has passed through the menopause period safely, without any of the symptoms so commonly associated with it."

VARICOSE VEINS

Varicose or enlarged veins may occur in any part of the body, but are usually found in the legs, where the circulation is more sluggish than in the upper part of the body. The walls of the veins become relaxed, and the veins themselves will often protrude, or will press inwardly upon the nerves of the leg sufficiently to cause quite painful symptoms. Ulcers may form on the vein, and these ulcers will exude a large amount of serum and finally blood.

Varicose veins are usually treated by surgery, where an entire section of the vein is removed, or the patient is advised to wear a rubber stocking (which makes the vein weaker and causes additional trouble).

Reportedly, varicose veins can be cured with rapid healing, rapid cleansing foods and a cleansing diet. A drugless doctor reports: "Local treatment of a beneficial kind may be used by the application several times a day of a piece of ice to the enlarged vein ... the ice pressed directly against the swollen part. This treatment should be continued from three to four minutes, during which time the muscles in the walls of the vein will become strengthened by the contraction produced by the ice ... treat at least twice daily, and as often as possible. ... Bear in mind the benefit to the whole circulatory system to be derived from living on a carefully selected diet. If varicose ulcers exist, they will disappear very rapidly during the fast.

"A woman, 73, had large varicose veins in the lower part of both legs, and several varicose ulcers. The pain was so great in both legs she could hardly walk. I immediately applied a strong treatment with the ultra-violet ray (from a mercury quartz generator), treating each ulcer for 20 seconds ... The patient was advised to take a plain water fast for four days, using two enemas daily. After this she was put on a general diet ... When she returned to my office (10 days later) I found that the ulcers were entirely healed, having been completely cured by the diet regimen and the one ultra-violet light treatment. All pain in the legs and the lower back had entirely disappeared, but there was still some enlargement of the veins in the legs. Accordingly, she was sent home with instructions to apply the treatment with ice...

"After another month she returned ... and an examination disclosed no signs of varicose veins. I advised her to apply the ice occasionally as a preventative treatment, and to remain on her well-balanced diet. That was three years ago, and the patient has had no return of either the varicose veins or the ulcers."

ANEMIA

A common name for this disease is often "green sickness," because of the fact that in the chronic form the skin turns a greenish sickly color. This condition is most common with young girls between the ages of 13 and 20. It may occur with either sex at any age.

In almost every case, another factor will be noticed, and that is constipation. Reportedly, in most cases, you will find a toxic state of the body induced by retention in the intestine, and also that excess acidity of the stomach is present. Other symptoms which are common are: great weakness, dizziness, headache, nausea, cold, clammy skin, ringing in the ears, feeble pulse, shortness of breath, pale tongue and nails and weak eyes.

If anyone has told you that you are anemic, do not be satisfied until you have had a blood examination. If anemia really exists, it is because of oxygen and iron starvation. Fasting can cure anemia, say some researchers, for the simple reason that the major cause of many cases is not actual lack of iron in food, but rather lack of power in the body to absorb it. While fasting, iron which has been stored in the body but not completely assimilated is taken up by the blood and used. In some cases the blood count actually doubles on a fast!

An osteopathic doctor reports: "Fasting on fruit is especially to be recommended for the first week, during which time the red corpuscles and hemoglobin will increase from 5 to 15 percent without any other treatment. This seems improbable at first thought, but has been proven by laboratory tests in hundreds of cases. ... During season, red cherries are the best fruit to use." This doctor tells of a young lady, 24, suffering from anemia. Her blood pressure was low, she suffered a valvular leakage of the heart, her skin was pale and anemic looking. A blood test showed only 50 percent of hemoglobin (she had only half as many red blood cells as normal, and this was true of her white blood cells, too).

She was put on an orange juice fast, taking the juice of one orange every two hours during the day, with a glass of water each time. Two enemas daily were advised, also two sponge baths. This fast was continued for one week, at the end of which time her hemoglobin had increased to 75 percent. For the next month, she used the following diet:

Breakfast—2 coddled eggs.
3 or 4 pieces of hard, thin, dry brown toast.
Dish of stewed fruit such as prunes, raisins, figs, apple sauce, baked apple.
Lunch— Raw apples, 2 ounces of pecan nuts, 1 glass of water.
Dinner— Lean beef.
2 nonstarchy vegetables, and a combination of salad vegetables.
Dessert: one of the stewed fruits as at breakfast and jello on alternate days—that is, fruit one day and jello the next.

After a month of this diet, her blood count was practically normal. She was then put on a general diet, and urged to use a large amount of blood-building foods, such as lean meat and salad and nonstarchy vegetables. The noon meal was changed from apples and nuts to a mixture of raw salad vegetables, with the addition of one starchy food. After several months, her blood tests were perfectly normal.

RAPID HEALING FOODS FOR HEART, VEINS AND ARTERIES!

Reportedly, spinach and nettle juices are effective in treating anemia. They are rich in iron and chlorophyll. These juices can be added to carrot juice. The dark-colored juices of grapes, beets and blueberries also help increase the production of red blood cells.

One medical doctor reports that high blood pressure cases must be put on a raw fruit diet, and little else. These fruits supply the blood and tissues with potassium, which helps to eliminate accumulated salt from the tissues. After three to four weeks, the blood pressure goes down to normal, in most cases. After three to four weeks on fruit or fruit juices, a normal diet should be resumed for at least six months. The best fruits to use are fresh apricots, peaches, cherries, pineapples, oranges and grapefruits. The best juices are citrus, black currants and grapes. "Works wonders," says this doctor. "Not only does the blood pressure come down, it stays down."

One rapid healing food in particular that has relieved heart, vein and artery problems is garlic. It has relieved high blood pressure in hundreds of cases, regardless of age or condition, often permanently, after prolonged use. No special diet need be followed, and it seemed safer and better than any drug. Garlic and onion dissolve the gooey sludge involved in hardening of the arteries, and may rid one of the build-up of fatty deposits on artery walls and help prevent arteries from clogging, say doctors. In one study, patients were simply served boiled or fried onions with breakfast or lunch. Garlic reduced cholesterol in test subjects who ate ¼ pound of butter below fasting level. In France, garlic and onions are used to dissolve blood clots in the legs of horses.

Wheat germ also contains a natural anti-clog ingredient, vitamin E, which has been used as follows: "For many years," says one woman, "I suffered from phlebitis, which eventually broke down and formed an ulcer, which would heal for a while, then break open again and again. After one severe case of infection, I had to have surgery, which helped, but only temporarily. By this time I had a great area of scar tissue which would crack, with the result, further ulceration occurred. My doctor wanted further surgery and skin graft, which I refused. I engaged a new doctor; he agreed with me a trial with vitamin E might be of some merit. He put me on 1600 units a day, plus application externally to the affected area. It was like magic. The ulcers healed, the scar tissue became pliable, no further breakage. The bulgy veins flattened down to normal. I stayed on vitamin E for six weeks under the doctor's supervision. Then decreased to 800 per day for three months. I now continue to take 400 units each day. Never felt better in my life."

A man says: "Last May I served on the election board ... and was on my feet practically all day. By the next morning an alarming blood clot had formed in the femoral vein in my left thigh. The flesh around the vein was red and inflamed. The vein stood out under the skin like a rope on the inside portion of my thigh and was very sore to the touch. I feared surgery. I had been taking about 1200 I.U. of vitamin E daily, so I decided to double the dose, and within 24 hours the clot began to disappear. The hard rope-like vein in my thigh had softened. I continued taking 2400 I.U. of vitamin E for several days. After five or six days the clot and inflammation had completely gone."

A medical journal reports that of 18 patients with Buerger's Disease treated with vitamin E, 17 were cured. A lady reports: "A few years ago, I suddenly developed Buerger's Disease in my left foot—the first three toes were cyanotic and I had an abscess on the third toe. I had terrific pains in my leg, painful walking, and was unable to sleep. I went to a doctor who wanted to amputate the toes. I refused. After reading about vitamin E, I immediately increased my intake from 800 I.U.'s daily to 1600 and gradually to 2400 I.U.'s a day, along with lecithin granules and 500 mg. of vitamin C—massaged my foot and exercised. Within three days the pain was almost gone and I was able to sleep and walk better. To say the least, I still have my toes and they look normal in color. I've always had a circulatory problem and three years ago dissolved a blood clot in my leg almost overnight with vitamin E."

Garlic may be extremely important in heart disorders, because it increases the absorption of thiamin (B-1) to 10 times the amount normally received from food or food supplements, an amount heretofore impossible to achieve except by liquid injection. Without B-1, heart muscles become weak and enlarged. A Harvard doctor has shown that an enlarged heart can be reduced in size in 48 hours with large doses of vitamin B-1, and another doctor recommends B-1 to all patients with indefinite heart symptoms. Rapid improvement follows, he says, and the heart is reduced in size.

For disorders in the normal heart function, juices of hawthorn and garlic can be added to other milder juices. Olive oil is healing to the heart. In one study in Greece, where olive oil is widely used, out of 1,214 men, only four cases of heart or artery disease were found in six years. It is said that soaking the feet for 10 minutes every day in a hot foot-bath prepared with shavings of castile soap (made with pure olive oil) can actually reduce cholesterol in the blood.

Papaya contains an enzyme called carpain, which seems helpful in heart ailments. For six months, one woman suffered extremely painful attacks of angina, and believed the end was near. She was advised to eat nothing but mangos and papaya. In a short time, her pains were completely gone, her heart beat normally and her health was restored. Another medical doctor reports that "in heart weakness I have found honey to have a marked effect in reviving heart action in keeping patients alive." For edema, or water-logged body tissues, fasting on watermelon, watercress, pears, peaches and nectarines may drain out pounds of fluid.

Simply drinking more fruit and vegetable juices is said to speed healing of leg ulcers. Onion and garlic may be added to carrot juice. Also effective are citrus and apple juices. A dressing of cabbage leaves and yellow onions over the ulcer speeds the healing process, says one researcher. Comfrey leaves are reported especially good for healing leg ulcers (mash and apply as a poultice just once a day).

QUICK RUNDOWN OF FOODS THAT HAVE BEEN USED IN TREATING SPECIFIC AILMENTS!

Anemia

apples
beef, lean
beets
blueberries
cherries, acerola
cherries, red
figs
garlic
grapes
honey
kelp
jello
liver
nettle tea
orange juice
prunes
raisins

Angina

lecithin
mangos
papaya

Circulation

citrus fruits
corn oil
lecithin
safflower oil
wheat germ

Edema (Swelling)

carrots
celery
nectarines
parsley
peaches
pears
pumpkin
watercress
watermelon

Hardening of Arteries

brewer's yeast
Brussels sprouts

garlic
kelp
lecithin
onion
peas
safflower oil
spinach, raw
soybean oil
tomatoes
wheat germ

Hemorrhage

blueberries
cherries, acerola
tomatoes

High Blood Pressure

apricots
asparagus
beans, string
beets

beet tops
brewer's yeast
carrots
celery
cherries
cucumber
currants
garlic
grapefruits
grapes
kale
kelp
lettuce
onions
orange
orange juice
oyster plant
parsley
parsnips
peaches
pineapple
spinach
squash, summer
Swiss chard
tomatoes
turnip
turnip tops

*Irregular Heart
Beat*
cherries, acerola

grapefruit juice

*Nausea,
Dizziness,
Tendency
Toward Little
Strokes*
lemon peel
lime peel
orange peel

Phlebitis
garlic
onion
wheat germ

Valvular Problems
apples
apricots
artichokes, fresh
asparagus
beans, string
beet tops
celery
cucumbers
eggplant
endive

figs
kale
lemon juice
lettuce
mustard greens
oyster plant
parsley
prunes
raisins
spinach
squash, summer
Swiss chard
tomatoes
turnip tops
watercress
wheat germ
zucchini

*Varicose Leg
Ulcers*
carrot juice
cabbage leaves
(dressing)
comfrey leaves
(dressing)
honey (dressing)
okra leaves
(dressing)
wheat germ

5

Rapid Healing Foods
for the Lungs!

During a cleansing diet, the gradual absorption of mucus from the miles of hair-like tubes in the lungs make deep and effortless breathing a most pleasant experience. The voice becomes clear and resonant. In some experiments, the volume of breath intake has doubled.

- Even severe cases of pneumonia can be cured by a cleansing diet. As one doctor reports, "Pneumonia in this way is not the serious thing at any age that we have come to consider it, and will yield as readily as any other so-called infection."

- The magic of the cleansing diet, says another doctor, will never be more quickly seen than when it relieves asthma! Advanced cases seem to yield as readily as those just beginning, he says—so do not think you are an exception because you have tried everything else, to no avail. "I do not know of a single case ... where the cure was not complete and permanent," he says.

- In cases of bronchitis, says this doctor, a cleansing diet will clear the lungs of accumulated material which has been forming for many years. A quick cure may be expected, he says!

Many a doctor advises a cleansing diet as the speediest way to get rid of a cold or the flu. One doctor suggests going on a cleansing raw fruit diet at the first sign of a cold—a diet consisting entirely of fruits or fruit juices—for two days. You may have all the fruit or fruit juices you wish, any variety. A person on a cleansing diet, he says, never catches a cold, and if you have one, it will rapidly clear up during a fruit fast. During a cleansing diet, germs are burned up or oxidized and eliminated and great quantities of mucus will be eliminated from the lungs.

AMAZING RECOVERY FROM PNEUMONIA

A medical doctor reports the case of a man who was taken with a severe cold, followed by a violent chill, high fever, pain, inability to breath sufficiently and a rapid development of catarrhal pneumonia. He was 60 years of age, and had weakened himself by overindulging in food and drink. Despite the best medical treatment, day after day he sank lower and was not expected to live. Other doctors had given him up and said he had only a few hours to live. His breathing was labored, his pulse barely audible.

This doctor, a medical man who did not believe in drugs, felt there was still hope, due to the enormous recuperative powers of the body when relieved of poisons. All drugs were immediately discontinued. The man was given an enema and other simple cleansing measures. In 15 minutes, his breathing became regular. The cyanosis was gone. In two hours, he was out of danger. The next morning he felt fine, but had no desire for food. In four days, he was back at work. Not for eight days did he feel the need to eat. By this time he was in the best health he had enjoyed since he was a young man.

"Other cases apparently as near death were saved in the same simple manner," says this doctor, "not by doing some heroic deed to prevent the impending death, but simply by relieving the body of much of its burden of intoxication quickly, with full reliance on the healing powers of Nature to restore a sick body to health if the impediments are removed."

BRONCHITIS

"This trouble," says one drugless doctor, "is really nothing more or less than a catarrhal state of the lungs, and all mucus forming foods must be eliminated until the delicate membrane (of the lungs) is restored to normal. A fast of several days will clear the lungs of accumulated material which has been forming for many years, and if a suitable diet is continued after the fasting period a quick cure may be expected."

This doctor reports the case of a man, 73, who had suffered for years from bronchitis. He thought he had asthma, because his lungs always made a whistling sound. He had tried to relieve his condition for years by using asthma remedies, and by various changes of climate, with little effect. Large quantities of mucus were coughed up each morning, and all during the day, in fact so much that he had trouble keeping a job. But his problem was only bronchitis, with excess mucus and waste in the lungs.

A fast of orange juice was prescribed, the patient taking the juice as desired during the day, and drinking plenty of water each time. After 15 days, a fruit fast was begun, and the patient used on successive days plums, grapes and apricots, using only one fruit on each day. By the end of the month (actually, sooner), the mucus had entirely disappeared, and the patient was not bringing up any more phlegm in the morning. He resumed a normal diet, but was told to cut down on carbohydrates.

In another case, an eight-year-old girl had suffered with bronchitis since infancy, with a bad cough and a whistling sound in the lungs. She had never been able to play with other children because her breath was so short. The cough became worse after her tonsils and adenoids were removed at age three (which frequently causes more mucus in the lungs).

After three days, drinking only orange juice and water, all signs of bronchitis disappeared, and no traces have since been found, using a practically starch-free, high protein diet, with a large amount of salad and green vegetables. She began taking dancing lessons, and was able to do the hardest exercises without the slightest fatigue, and without producing any whistling or wheezing in the lungs.

ASTHMA

Asthma is not an allergy, says one drugless doctor. When

cured with this method, an allergy sufferer can *bathe* in pollen without any ill effects. And the same is true of foods, cats or anything else. They will have no effect on you once you are cured with this method. The elimination of poisons in the respiratory tract results in a permanent clearing up of symptoms and the individual no longer suffers from asthma, he says. "As no other means of care results in a more rapid freeing of the body of its toxic load ... nothing brings relief from asthma as certainly and speedily as the fast," he says. "Usually within 24 to 36 hours the worst cases are enabled to lie flat in their beds and to breathe easily and sleep ... after several days the secretion of mucus will cease."

Relief is permanent, says another doctor. "Asthmatics suffer year after year, often becoming worse, when all of them could get well in four to eight weeks and remain so the rest of their lives," he says. "Thousands have done so."

Difficulty in breathing, a struggle to draw enough air into the lungs, resulting in the peculiar wheeze of the asthma victim attempting to inhale, are the most characteristic symptoms of asthma.

Reportedly, a permanent cure depends entirely upon the following—

1. The development of a strong diaphragm, so the patient can inhale and exhale to the extreme with perfect freedom of movement.
2. Avoiding those foods which produce an excess of stomach and intestinal gas, until digestion is improved to the point where properly proportioned meals may be taken. The complete fast should be used at the start of the cure if you wish to see the wheezing stop in from 12 to 48 hours.

"The magic of the fast will never be more quickly seen than in its application to this malady," says one drugless doctor. "Advanced cases yield as readily as those just beginning."

A young man, 34, had been subject to asthmatic attacks since childhood, and had not been able to either play ball or climb hills at any time of his life. He smoked asthmatic cigarettes all day long, and kept asthmatic powders burning in his room most of the night. He had been doing this for several years, and seemed to be getting worse each year.

With this method, he was put on a complete fast for 20 days, using only water in whatever quantities desired. In order to relieve him quickly of the accumulated fecal matter in his colon, he was immediately given 3 ounces of castor oil mixed with 4 ounces of lemon juice. This, together with the enemas which he started taking, flushed the colon so completely of feces and gas, that he was able to sleep clear through the night on the very first night after starting treatment.

Then the following diet was prescribed, for the next 10 days:

Breakfast—Whites of 3 eggs.
        3 pieces of hard, thin, dry, brown toast.
        5 stewed prunes.

Lunch— 1 of the following medium-starch vegetables: carrots, turnips, parsnips, beets.
        2 nonstarchy vegetables.
        1 salad vegetable.

Dinner— A choice of 1 of the following: lean beef or chicken.
        A choice of 2 nonstarchy vegetables.
        1 salad vegetable.

In about a month, the patient was so recovered that he was able to climb Mount Wilson, Mount Lowe and Camp Baldy, three of the highest points in Southern California, on successive days. His lungs were entirely free from any tendency to wheeze, and the trouble has never reappeared since at any time of the day or night (for six years), avoiding gas-producing foods. He can now even eat gassy foods, by combining them with other foods (nonstarchy) which counter the effect, relieving pressure on the diaphragm, which caused his trouble in the first place.

A six-year-old boy had been troubled with asthmatic wheezing since a few days after birth, brought about by constant gas pressure. His abdomen was distended, and the wheezing kept him awake every night. With this method, the mother was told to give the child only small amounts of orange juice and water (using in all about six oranges daily) for three and a half days. An enema was given the first day, at about mid-afternoon and another about 8 o'clock at night, and the child slept through the entire night for the first time in his life. Since then he has slept 11 or 12 hours every night.

After the fast the following diet was given—

Breakfast—Whites of 2 eggs.
        2 pieces of brown toast softened in hot water and seasoned with butter.
        3 stewed unsulphured prunes.

Lunch— Dish of cottage cheese.
Dish of cooked spinach or celery.
1 piece of toast softened as at breakfast.
Dinner— 1 small piece of steak.
1 nonstarchy vegetable.
1 salad vegetable.

To guard against the possibility of any asthmatic attack during the night, an enema was used each night before the child was put to bed, but this was soon discontinued, as it was apparent in a very few days that there would be no return of the gas pressure. This diet was kept up for several months, and the child is now eating normally (a well-balanced diet).

An 82-year-old Army veteran had suffered with asthma ever since the war, and had been living for many years in a Soldier's Home—much of the time confined to bed. He had been unable to work because of asthma, and had lived on a pension almost entirely, except for any help his children could provide.

He was put on an orange juice fast, taking a glass of orange juice three times daily, with a glass of water each time. He continued this fast for about 25 days. After the second day all signs of asthmatic wheezing disappeared, and after about the twentieth day the mucus discharges which he had coughed up for years entirely disappeared, and his lungs were as clear as if there had never been any trouble. He continued living at the same home, in perfect health for a man his age, without a trace of asthma.

RAPID HEALING FOODS FOR THE LUNGS!

Berries, fresh pineapple, tomatoes, lemons, oranges, grapefruits, limes, strawberries and most sour fruits tend to dissolve accumulations of mucus in the system. They should be eaten on an exclusively raw fruit diet, says one drugless doctor. Mashed cranberries, strained and mixed with warm water, are said to stop asthmatic wheezing and cause an almost immediate opening of the bronchial tubes, just like adrenalin. Here is a breakdown of specific foods that may be used for specific lung problems (starred items are those which seem especially helpful):

Asthma

Apples*
Apricots
Cabbage
Carrots
Cauliflower
Cherries*
Comfrey tea*
Cranberries*
Endives
Garlic*
Guava
Lemon juice*
Nectarines
Onion
Oranges*
Peppers (green)
Raisins (stewed
   juice)
Tangerines*
Turnip greens
Water in which
   turnip roots are
   boiled

Bronchitis

Apples*
Apricots
Dates
Elderberry*
Garlic*
Leeks*
Mustard greens
Onion*
Oranges*
Peaches
Pineapples*
Plums
Rhubarb
Spinach
Tangerines*
Turnip greens

Emphysema

Grapes and*
Grape juice
   (see also
   Bronchitis)

Pneumonia

Grapefruit*

Kumquats*
Lemon juice*
Onion*
Oranges*
Tangerines

Pleurisy

Grape juice*
Persimmons
Onion (crushed,
   applied
   to chest as
   a poultice)*
Okra

Flu

Garlic*
Leeks
Onions*

Fevers

Lemon*
Mango*
Oranges
Tangerines

Garlic dissolves mucus in the sinuses, bronchial tubes and lungs. It is the most powerful natural antibiotic known in pure food. It can kill cold, flu and virus germs in 10 minutes. It cuts phlegm, fights infections, clears sinuses, bronchial tubes and lungs. In cases of asthma, bronchitis and emphysema, one researcher reports 90 percent of such sufferers quickly relieved or cured. It has made lung abscesses vanish. It does not even have to be eaten. Its ethers are so potent and penetrating they dissolve mucus when inhaled. One woman stated: "It was from an herb book that I learned about the wonders of garlic, and it cleared up pneumonia congestion in my lungs when antibiotics failed."

It is called poor man's penicillin. Reportedly, 1 milligram of this plant equaled 25 units of penicillin. It even fights some germs penicillin won't touch. Unlike penicillin, available only in doctor-prescribed drugs that may cause serious side effects or allergic reaction, this plant is safe and available without prescription, and can be eaten for enjoyment. Its germ-killing power remains in the bloodstream for 10 hours.

Vinegar also has germ-cleansing power, and can heal the lungs. An inexpensive vinegar vapor method—in a vaporizer, place 2 tablespoonfuls of vinegar in a quart of boiling water, and inhale 15 minutes three times a day—can be used in the home for patients with chronic pulmonary suppuration (lung infection with pus), says one medical doctor. It has accomplished what penicillin could not.

Honey is rapid cleansing food for the lungs. It has a fatal effect on germs, due to its moisture absorbing ability. When germs come in contact with honey, all their moisture is withdrawn—they shrivel and die. It relieves inflammation and soothes painful coughing spasms. It even relieved pneumonia, with actual penicillin power. A young girl was given up to die. Doctors said she had a hopeless case of TB. Someone suggested a diet of honey and goat's milk, and she was soon cured. At 90 she was still spry. At a time when TB was considered the nation's number one killer (they called it the White Plague), a man who came down with it was given only a few weeks to live. Doctors said flatly his lungs were so mottled he could not be cured. He began using honey daily. Five years later, his lungs were so healthy, the doctors refused to believe it was him!

Grape juice is said to have miraculous powers in clearing up mucus and phlegm. One drugless doctor recommends it for pleurisy and emphysema. In severe cases, he says, eat nothing except undiluted, unsweetened grape juice, as much as desired, for three or four weeks (grapes may be eaten as well). In less severe cases, he recommends a meat and grape juice diet. White chicken meat, without the skin, and lean meats (especially steak or veal), are recommended. These should be baked, broiled or stewed. Any grape juice may be used, but Concord grapes are best, he says. Diabetics may not be able to use this method, and should check with their doctor first, he says. The grape juice seems to cleanse the blood of poisons. This doctor says he recovered from a collapsed right lung with this method, says nothing else worked as well and that it gives him amazing energy.

He tells of a patient, in her late sixties, with an advanced case of emphysema, and very labored breathing: 500 cc was all she could exhale. With this diet, in one week she was exhaling 2,000 cc, an improvement of 300 percent. He reports another case of advanced emphysema, a mine worker, 63, who had a bloated belly due to labored breathing. He followed the diet faithfully, and his breathing improved rapidly—in fact, his bloated belly lost 1 inch per day, every day for a week![1]

---

[1]*Old Fashioned Health Remedies That Work Best*, by L.L. Schneider, D.C., N.D. (Parker Publishing Company, Inc., West Nyack, N.Y.), 1977.

6

Rapid Healing Food for Liver and Gall Bladder!

The liver is a gland situated on the right side of the body. It acts as a filter to purify the blood, and secretes bile through the gall bladder, into the stomach. (Bile is needed to break up fatty and oily foods.) When the liver becomes lazy or congested, or the bile duct inflamed for any reason, bile does not flow freely, may become impacted (forming stones), and poisons accumulate in the system. Food, especially fat, is not digested completely, and vitamins A, D, E and K are not absorbed. This, of course, can lead to circulatory problems, problems with sugar metabolism, skin problems—and it frequently causes eye weakness.

High fat intake can overburden your liver with wastes, impairing liver function, interfering with circulation, depriving the liver of needed oxygen, choking liver cells and clogging them with fat.

Signs that the liver is bogged down with accumulated poisons include headache, nausea, indigestion, loss of appetite, constipation, pain on the right side, especially after fatty foods, a jaundiced or yellowed skin, cold sweats, a frequent belching bitter taste, heart-attack, heartburn or ulcer symptoms, gas, a feeling of fullness or bloating after meals, and in general many of the same symptoms associated with gall bladder trouble.

REMEDY FOR A SLUGGISH LIVER

When these symptoms persist, it is an indication that bile is being stored up in the liver and not sufficiently eliminated. Some common causes are:

1. **Eating more food of every kind than the body can use.**
2. **Bad habits other than eating, which waste energy that should be used by the liver: drinking, smoking, late hours, excesses of every kind.**
3. **Constipation and internal toxemia due to the reabsorption of poisons which have not been expelled rapidly enough.**
4. **A sluggish liver produces depression and is caused by it— i.e., depression causes stagnation of the biliary fluids.**
5. **Another cause is often the stoppage of the bile ducts by catarrhal inflammation of the ducts, causing stricture; also the pressure caused by pregnancy, and by the lodgment of gallstones which may stop the flow.**

The cure is not difficult, say drugless doctors. Certain foods, such as sugars, starches, fats like butter, eggs and cream, spices, alcohol and chocolate, should be avoided for a while, and this will bring about very satisfactory results.

But the cure is rapid if a fruit fast is strictly adhered to for a few days, say these doctors. This should be followed by careful dieting until the liver is able to do a reasonable amount of work.

One such doctor states: "Clinical experience and observation have shown beyond the shadow of a doubt that large doses of olive oil, combined with an equal amount of the juice of some citrus fruit, such as the orange, lemon or grapefruit, will dissolve the thickened bile and aid in bringing about quick results in patients suffering from any form of inorganic liver trouble." (The exact dosage and time for taking are described in detail on pages 103-104.) This doctor reports the following case.

A young lady, 34, had suffered headaches for years, which could only be relieved by a certain medicine—which she had taken until the liver did not seem to function properly without this drug. Ordinary headache remedies had no effect. Missing a meal would always bring on a severe sick headache, making it necessary for her to stay home from work, and remain in bed in a darkened room.

This doctor promised her that her headaches would vanish forever, if she would follow this method for 10 days: fast on water with a glass of orange juice three times daily. It worked so well, she was able to return to work the next day. At the end of 10 days, her sallow skin had cleared, her eyeballs were again white, and she felt the return of her best physical and mental powers. Afterward, she was told to eat more greens and salad vegetables, exercise more and take enemas daily until her intestines were able to function normally. She has remained in the best of health ever since, and for over two years has had no more headaches.

During this time, her mother took almost the same identical treatment, and was cured of migraine headaches, which she had since a small child. (The cause of all so-called sick headaches, says this doctor, is toxemia or internal poisoning of the body by its own wastes.)

HOW GALLSTONES MAY VANISH
WITHOUT SURGERY!

Gallstones begin with excess bile produced by the liver, in response to large amounts of greasy, fatty, fried foods, pastry and sweets. The excess bile, having nowhere to go, remains in the gall bladder (a storage pouch under the liver), and may even back up. Continual stimulation and congestion leads to irritation and inflammation of the gall bladder—which, in effect, becomes swollen and sluggish. In this state, it cannot empty completely as bile is needed. Without bile (a bitter green fluid), food in the stomach is not fully digested, and eventually becomes impacted in the colon, resulting in constipation.

In the bowels, fermenting and putrefying material is reabsorbed into the blood—which passes on to the liver for purification. When the liver has more poisons than it

can handle (from an overstuffed colon), the bile it
secretes is impure, which leads to gall bladder infection, with pus and germs.

The medical treatment of gall bladder infections and gallstones consists of a low-fat diet, special bile tablets and, in
advanced cases, artificial drainage of the gall bladder or its
complete removal. The patient is immediately relieved and goes
back to his old eating habits—and gall bladder symptoms
return, even after surgery (such cases are helped, say drugless
doctors, with these methods).

Drugless doctors claim:

- **There is no need to operate for gallstones. Too many
  organs are removed that could be saved by draining them
  with a simple cleansing diet.**
- **Instead of surgically draining the gall bladder, a cleansing
  diet will enable the body to perform an excellent job of
  drainage and do it in a way to leave the gall bladder intact
  and unharmed.**
- **A cleansing diet restores normal liver function so that bile
  chemistry becomes normal again—and normal bile will
  dissolve these stones. The sand will pass into the intestines
  and be eliminated.**

A medical doctor who treated hundreds of gallstones without surgery stated: "Given proper assistance, the chemistry of
the body can be so altered that stones soften, disintegrate and
pass out with but slight discomfort. We have treated many cases
and seldom have we found it necessary to resort to surgery. It is a
remarkable fact that this softening occurs very rapidly (on a
cleansing diet—in 8 to 10 days)."

This doctor was referring to a complete fast, but says that for
people who suffer recurrent attacks there is no treatment in the
intervals to equal a diet of fresh fruits, salads and cooked
nonstarchy vegetables, exclusively.

To this, another doctor added: "Reform the diet ... At the
same time empty the colon thoroughly every day by means of the
2-quart cool enema, and the worst cases of pus gall bladder will
recover. They must recover. In my experience they always have
done so, simply because the causes of the various infections and
irritations of this organ are removed and kept continually
removed by these very simple means."

Drugless doctors say that simple gall bladder and bile duct infection is completely remedied on fasts of one to three weeks' duration. The pus is removed, the inflammation subsides and the tissues are healed during this physiological rest. Stones are softened and later disintegrate and pass into the bowels. With the removal of the stones, all pain ceases and recovery is complete and permanent with this method, they say.

RAPID RELIEF CLAIMED!

One doctor claimed that fully one-half of the patients who came to him believing they had stomach ulcers or gastritis, had gall bladder trouble. Using only rapid cleansing foods and a cleansing diet, he claimed: "I have found a very large number of cases ... which have responded so rapidly ... as to lose all symptoms in a day or two.

"I have had many cases where large gallstones have been removed by my treatment, where no typical gallstone colic had been experienced at all. If the sharp pains and contractions of the gallstone colic are present in their worst form, the patient will be unable to stand or even sit up straight, but will be forced to lie down with the knees drawn up to the chest. Even this position does not relieve the pain. I am convinced that these colicky symptoms are not present in most cases, and that a serious stoppage of bile or a blocking up of the bile ducts with a gallstone may be present without any of such symptoms being in evidence at all.

"There is no doubt that this disorder is caused by overindulgence in starches and sugars, without sufficient vigorous exercise to take care of the excess. Out of thousands of cases of this trouble which have come under my observation, I have never discovered one affecting an athlete ... It occurs almost entirely among those living a sedentary life, and who insist on eating such a kind and quantity of food as only hard physical exercise would necessitate.

"The first method of treatment to be used for any disorder of the liver or gall bladder is the olive oil and fruit juice regime. **Caution: use only if your doctor has determined with x-rays that your gallstones are small enough to pass without getting stuck, and gives his approval.** Just before retiring, the patient usually takes 4 ounces of olive oil, together with 4 ounces of lemon, orange or grapefruit juice. The oil and fruit juice are beaten up well together into as much of an emulsion as possible, and the mixture, if taken just before retiring, is less liable to cause nausea while the patient is asleep. This may be taken on one night only, or on several nights in succession, and should be followed by a fast with grapefruit juice, lemon juice or orange juice. This fast should be continued as long as necessary, and the olive oil treatment may be taken as many times as seems advisable to accomplish a thorough cleansing of the gall bladder and liver. ...

"After the removal of the gallstones has been accomplished, do not forget that an increased amount of exercise is absolutely essential to ensure a permanent cure. The carbohydrates must be reduced in quantity (permanently)." This doctor reported the following case.

200 STONES PASSED!

A man, 50, had suffered from a number of gall bladder attacks, and had been told he needed surgery, but would not consent, because in several cases he knew—where operations had been performed—the patients had only received temporary relief, and afterward had a more aggravated form of trouble than before.

"I was called in on the case," said this doctor, "while he was having a most severe attack of gallstone colic. ... At first he was so nauseated that everything taken into his stomach would be immediately vomited, and the olive oil regime could not be administered until after the acute attack had subsided. However, through the use of small amounts of lemon juice, together with hot applications over the gall bladder and hot enemas, the trouble was sufficiently relieved during the first day to enable him ... to retain 4 ounces of olive oil and 4 ounces of lemon juice. After taking these he was able to sleep for 12 hours, being utterly exhausted from the acute attack.

"As soon as he awakened he was given an enema of 2 quarts of hot water. This brought away about 200 small gallstones with quantities of bile and mucus. The olive oil treatment was administered each night for three more days, the patient using a lemon juice fast during the rest of the time; that is, taking the juice of half a lemon in a glass of water every half-hour of the day. The fast was not continued long, as the patient wanted to get back to his office for some important business, so he was put upon a careful diet, and the olive oil and grapefruit juice taken every third day for six more times. The bilestones and gallstones continued to come out with the enemas until they were all gradually eliminated, and at the end of 30 days there was no further sign of anything except bile being brought away.

"This cure was effected over four years ago, and the patient has remained in perfect health ever since, with not the slightest return of any symptom of gallstones. He has also remained well in every way, without any of the headaches which he experienced for so many years, and which were no doubt caused by a chronic state of biliousness." Here is another amazing case from this doctor's files.

OVERNIGHT RELIEF!

A woman, 71, with liver and gall bladder trouble seemed to have a large amount of gallstones. She refused to believe it, as it only seemed like indigestion and stomach trouble. However, she was soon convinced.

The first night under treatment, she took the grapefruit juice and olive oil regime, following this with a fast of grapefruit juice, taking the juice of a grapefruit every two hours, with a glass of water. The first morning—on moving her bowels (with the aid of an enema)—she eliminated a large quantity of gallstones. Her digestion was improved and she felt better in every way for about three weeks. Then gall bladder symptoms returned briefly. She went to the bathroom and eliminated a large gallstone about 1¼" in diameter. This large stone came out without any cramps or colic.

"This cure," said the doctor, "was completed over a year ago, and the patient has remained perfectly well since that time, having lost entirely all of the digestive disorders from which she had suffered for years. She declares that she does not know of any time in her life when she felt so well as at present. She is living on a simple, well-selected diet, but even at such times as she has used prohibited foods she has felt no distress whatsoever."

RAPID HEALING FOODS
FOR THE LIVER!

Reportedly, apples stimulate all body secretions. They contain malic and tartaric acids which help prevent liver trouble. Cherries and dandelion greens are very cleansing to the liver. Grapefruit, parsley, pomegranate, quince, raspberries, strawberries, tangerines and tomatoes help relieve a sluggish liver and liver congestion. Watercress relieves inflammation of the liver. Here is a complete list of foods that have been used to relieve liver problems:

apple juice	dandelion tea	pomegranate
apples	endives	quince
artichokes	gooseberries	radish juice
beet juice	garlic	raspberries
beet leaves, boiled	grapefruit	sesame seeds
carrot juice	grape juice	spinach
carrots	grapes	strawberries
cauliflower	lemon juice	tangerines
cherries	olive oil	tomatoes
collards	olives	turnip greens
cranberries	orange juice	walnuts
dandelion greens	peppers, green	watercress
	plums	

Dandelion tea (a strong cupful twice a day) seems to cleanse and purify the liver. One doctor claimed to have relieved liver problems in almost every case, including his own, with this tea. For him, it was the only thing that worked after 15 years of misery. His nurse recommended it.

Garlic's major value in liver disorders is its power to detoxify putrefactive bacteria in the intestines, and thereby give the liver a rest (it is the liver that cleanses blood coming up from the intestines). It is an aid to increased and vigorous circulation through the liver. It is claimed that a teaspoon of garlic (diced) mixed with a tablespoon of olive oil or soybean oil, taken at night will liven up the liver and so rejuvenate it that the skin of the body will glow with renewed vitality.

Grapes help combat liver disorders, jaundice and stimulate bile flow. They have been recommended to relieve a sluggish liver, with pain or tenderness on the right side—in a meat and grape juice diet (white chicken meat without the skin or lean meat like steak or veal), no other food or drink, as long as necessary. Grapes may be eaten, as well. Diabetics should not use this.

RAPID HEALING FOODS
FOR THE GALL BLADDER!

In general, the same foods used for liver problems, will reportedly help gall bladder sufferers. Here is a list of specific foods that have been used to relieve gall bladder problems:

apple juice	dandelion tea	parsley tea
apricots	endives	pears
barley water	gooseberries	radish juice
beet juice	grains, unrefined	rhubarb
beet leaves, boiled	grapefruit	rose petal tea
beet tops	grapefruit juice	soybean lecithin
bran	grape juice	squash
Brewer's yeast	lemon juice	sunflower seeds
carrot juice	nuts	vinegar
chamomile tea	olive oil	walnuts
dandelion greens	orange juice	water

Apples contain malic and tartaric acids, said to be of great value in dissolving out gallstones and gravel from the urinary organs. The same is true of rose petal tea. Plain, boiled beet leaves have been found to clear the bile duct of its clogging debris. Eat a large portion and nothing else that day, says one doctor. Beet tops are also said to speed the flow of bile. Bran and other high fiber cereals start the bile juice flowing, and sweep degenerated bile salts out of the colon. They are a good way to start the day, and most patients report relief of symptoms, say doctors.

More fluid intake is also recommended, especially water. The best juices to use in treating gall bladder inflammation are grape, carrot and beet, with small additions of dandelion and radish juice, says one researcher. Pear juice is also very effective in relieving gall bladder trouble. Chamomile tea has dissolved gallstones in as little as 24 hours. Lemon juice is so powerful it can stimulate, purge and empty the gall bladder, says one doctor, who recommends 3 tablespoons of undiluted unsweetened lemon juice, 15 to 30 minutes before breakfast daily, for a week.

Reportedly, lemon juice also helps to relieve the nausea gall bladder victims may suffer.

Mrs. S.W. recalled: "Shortly after the birth of my baby, I had a very painful attack under my right ribs. After many days of tests, lots of pain-killers and several more attacks, the x-rays showed gallstones. The doctors wanted to remove my gall bladder as soon as possible, stating it was the only way to take care of the problem. They assured me I didn't really need my gall bladder anyway. A day before the operation was scheduled, I cancelled it. A girlfriend took me to a different doctor who treated ailments naturally. He recommended virgin olive oil, starting with 1 tablespoon and working up to ¼ cup in grapefruit juice every morning first thing. In three weeks I worked up to the quarter cup and stopped. It must have been long enough, because I no longer have attacks. It's been over a year."

One woman, scheduled for gallstone surgery, tried this method: take 4 tablespoons of olive oil with the juice of ½ lemon an hour before breakfast each day. She did this for six months and found no need for surgery.

One doctor claims you can usually get a lazy gall bladder into action by simply taking 1 or 2 tablespoons of olive oil before each meal. This starts the flow of bile before the rest of the food enters the stomach. You may experience some indigestion the first few days, but you'll see a marked improvement in two weeks, he says. Olive oil seems to dissolve gallstones. In one experiment, a gallstone lost 69 percent of its weight in two days when immersed in pure olive oil. Doctors report it causes strong contractions of the gall bladder, and induces complete emptying. Olive oil tends to expand the duct through which gallstones must pass, says one doctor. It lubricates the lining of the duct and makes it sufficiently slippery to let the stones slide out painlessly, he says.

One method of passing gallstones (see page 103) is to mix ½ cup olive oil with ½ cup lemon or grapefruit juice, stir and drink, then go to bed. In the morning, drink something hot, and you may pass the stones from your bowels. Another method is to fast two days, drink apple juice every two hours and use the above method (same caution) on the second night. One man with five gallstones who used this method fasted three days on apple juice, and then drank ½ cup olive oil with ½ cup apple juice on the third night. He says his gallstones passed on the fourth day.

Vinegar has been used to relieve gall bladder pain. One woman wrote: "My husband and I both were bothered with gall bladder pains for about a year. When talking with a naturopath he told us to take, first thing in the morning before anything else, 1 ounce of vegetable oil and follow with 4 ounces of grapefruit juice...we substituted 4 ounces of water with a teaspoon of vinegar. We were never bothered again with any pains...a year later we ran out of oil and did not use any for three weeks. The gall bladder pains returned, but immediately left as soon as we started the oil and vinegar water again. Now another year has gone and we are still not bothered with gall bladder pains."

Squash is extremely high in vitamin A (4,950 I.U. per 100 grams). Experiments have proven that foods high in vitamin A dissolve gallstones and prevent them from forming. Parsley, also high in vitamin A, is excellent to help relieve a congested liver and gall bladder. Other foods that help cleanse and empty a congested gall bladder include grapefruit, gooseberries, endives and dandelion greens (which are also helpful in cleansing the spleen).

Lecithin, a fat-dissolver produced by the body, and available in foods, seems to liquefy cholesterol, an important substance in gallstones. Among the foods high in lecithin are soybeans and sunflower seeds. Foods that stimulate increased production of lecithin by the body are Brewer's yeast, nuts (especially walnuts) and unrefined grains. These foods, therefore, help prevent gallstones, for the thickened, gritty, impure and coagulating bile, stagnating in a swollen gall bladder, forming stones, is dissolved by lecithin.

7

Rapid Healing Foods for Kidneys, Bladder and Urinary Organs!

Inflammation of the kidneys is caused by the most irritating and destructive of all poisons—nitrogenous waste. Ordinarily, this poisonous waste does not cause trouble. But it builds up from excessive eating, and continual irritation from spicy foods, alcoholic beverages, soft drinks, chocolates, sugars and starches. This sets up an inflammation of the lining membrane of the kidneys (called nephritis or Bright's disease).

Kidney inflammation is deadly and painful. It starts with traces of albumen in the urine. The urine will gradually become cloudy and often scant, and pain will develop in the back and lower spine because of the irritation produced in the kidneys and bladder from this heavy, irritating urine.

Granular bloody sediment may appear in the urine, with headaches, vertigo, frequent urges, night rising and scanty urine. The urine smells bad, as well. In advanced cases, there is a backup of urinary waste that causes swelling or bloating of the body, called dropsy (or edema). To cure kidney inflammation, just stop causing it, say drugless doctors. Eat less concentrated foods, and more rapid cleansing foods, like fresh juicy fruits and leafy vegetables. A medical doctor who pioneered in the use of cleansing foods says: "By the use of raw, unprocessed and uncooked foods you will greatly hasten recovery."

RAPID RELIEF CLAIMED!

A little girl, age 10, was doomed with nephritis. Doctors told her parents she had only a month to live. She was bloated from head to foot with water (dropsy). "Nothing can be done," they all said. Then a drugless doctor was called. "Yes, I believe she can be helped," he said. The child was put to bed, on a fast: no food, only small sips of water, from time to time.

Almost overnight, the swelling disappeared—pounds of water were drained away—her elephant-sized wrists and ankles became normal. In two weeks, food was resumed. First, juicy fruits and leafy vegetables, and after a few days, starches, sugars and proteins were added.

In nine months she was considered cured. She grew up, the picture of radiant health—no more kidney trouble—in fact, she was never ill at all, and led a busy, active life. This case reveals the amazing way the body can regenerate itself, if given a chance, with a cleansing diet.

- **"There is no disease which yields so readily to treatment (by a cleansing diet) as this one, and even the most serious looking cases will often be cured in a remarkably short time ... (Irreversible) cases are very rare ... a complete cure can usually be effected," says one drugless doctor.**

- **Another doctor says: "There is no chronic disease that so quickly improves, and from which the patient is so likely to make a full recovery (in all but the most advanced cases)."**

Ten days, two weeks, sometimes three, is all it takes, he says. The kidneys quickly clear up. Albumen disappears from the urine, casts and blood clear up. The symptoms of urine poisoning, headaches, vertigo, frequent urination, bedwetting, frequent night rising, scanty urine—soon cease. The urine becomes normal.

ANOTHER AMAZING RECOVERY!

A doctor reports the following case. A man, 42, suffering from kidney inflammation for eight years, was hardly able to attend to business, and felt that he had "reached the end of the line" as he put it. He had high blood pressure (180 mm, which is 6 mm above normal), and large amounts of albumen in his urine. He had been turned down for life insurance, repeatedly, on account of this ailment.

He had learned to examine his urine by boiling it in a test tube, and after heating, the coagulated albumen was so heavy that it could not be poured out. This doctor immediately put him on a cleansing diet—using one particular food, a delicious sweet fruit.

He was told to use as many grapes as desired during the day, and drink large quantities of water. Nothing else, no other food or drink. His method was to eat a handful of grapes whenever he felt like it at any time of day, limiting himself only to the extent of not taking more than 3 pounds on any given day.

In four days, his urine was entirely clear of any signs of albumen. At the end of a week, his blood pressure had returned to normal (120 mm). He was then told to fast on fruit or fruit juices for the rest of the month (a glass of orange juice three times a day, with a glass of water each time, for a week; then an apple fast, using a small, juicy apple every two hours, with a glass of water, for the rest of the month). Then he was placed on the following diet:

Soup to be taken three times daily, made from the following vegetables: spinach, asparagus, celery, parsley. These were ground together in a food grinder, and cooked for about two hours.

He was allowed to use as much of this as he desired three times a day, and encouraged to drink a large amount of water between meals. This special diet was used for four days, after which time he was given the following:

Breakfast—Whites of 3 eggs.
>> 3 or 4 pieces of thin, dry, brown toast.
>> Dish of stewed fruit, selected from the following: prunes, figs, raisins, dried apricots.
Lunch— 2 ounces of almond or pecan nuts.
>> 2 or 3 apples.
Dinner— One-half pound Salisbury steak.
>> 2 nonstarchy vegetables.
>> Choice of one or more salad vegetables.
>> Dessert: every other day a dish of stewed fruit and on the alternate days a dish of jello, with whipped cream if desired.

No drugs were used. "This cure was effected more than six years ago," the doctor stated, "and the patient has remained in perfect health ever since, without any return of high blood pressure. Of course he has followed his diet during these years, has learned more about selecting food and has never returned to his former habit of indiscriminate eating."

KIDNEY STONES DISSOLVE RAPIDLY!

Kidney stone pain has been described as the most excruciating pain the body can endure. The first symptoms which will be felt when a stone has formed will be sharp, shooting pains from one side or the other, around the back to the bladder, that refuse to go away.

The stones, themselves, consist of various wastes which solidify in the urine and become massive crystals often hard enough to cut glass. "I have handled many cases," says one drugless doctor, "and have never been forced to recommend surgical intervention. I have found that in every case (with a cleansing diet), the kidney stone may be dissolved sufficiently, so that the pieces will pass down the ureter into the bladder, and finally out..."

A cleansing fruit juice diet (and nothing else, no other food or drink), which he recommends, "seems to have a specific effect in dissolving the (kidney stones) ... I find it frequently the case that the kidney stone will be dissolved into such minute particles that there will not be any pain as these particles pass through the body ... (These cleansing foods) seem to dissolve the stone so finely that no irritation is produced." This doctor reports the following case.

A man, 50, was having a severe kidney stone attack, and was in excruciating agony. He was under heavy sedation. A number of doctors had declared his case incurable without an operation, believing that the stone was so large it could not be dissolved. This man was immediately told to fast on lemon juice (½ lemon to a glass of water), every half hour. In a few hours, the pain subsided enough for him to come for an x-ray—which revealed the size of the stone. He was advised to continue this cleansing diet for a few days (no other food or drink), and all kidney pains disappeared in five days. The doctor says:

"The fast was continued for five more days, and the patient then put on a general diet. Of course hot enemas were used several times daily during this fast, and the patient was encouraged to drink an extra amount of hot water over and above the regular doses of lemon juice and hot water each half hour."

At the end of three weeks, when x-rays were taken, the stone was gone. "There have been no symptoms since that time, now almost a year ago, and the patient has remained well in every way." This doctor stresses that a large amount of water must be used, with the addition of lemon juice (½ lemon to a glass) to avoid pain.

KIDNEY ABSCESS DRAINED!

Other doctors report similar results. Dr. Otto Buchinger, who used cleansing diets successfully in 30,000 cases, reports that his first patient, a woman physician, aborted a handful of kidney stones after 11 days. Dr. Herbert Shelton, another great advocate of cleansing diets, reports that a case of kidney abscess—that is, infection with pus—which other doctors diagnosed as a stone requiring surgery, was completely drained with a cleansing diet, a 4-ounce glass full of pus passing all at one time.

BLADDER INFLAMMATION
(Cystitis)

In acute inflammation of the bladder pain will frequently be felt when the bladder is full of urine, and also immediately after it is emptied. As the walls of the bladder collapse with no urine to hold them apart, one side will rub against the other, producing a shooting pain not only in the bladder itself but up either side of the groin, to the lower spine. The most common cause of bladder inflammation is irritating substances in the urine which inflame the lining of the bladder or urethra, the passage leading out of the body.

No matter what kind of irritating material exists in the urine, says one doctor, it can be eliminated with a cleansing diet, using one particular cleansing food: water. Expect to be entirely free from these pains, says this doctor, when the bladder is healed of all inflammation. In addition, hot sitz baths are recommended (sit in about 9 inches of hot water with only the hips and feet immersed). Reportedly, women will find that several hot douches a day will aid in relieving the symptoms, until the lining of the bladder is completely healed. In an acute attack, relief can be obtained by lying on the back with the hips elevated. Urinating while leaning far forward helps to completely empty the bladder, without any afterflow. Reportedly, heat applications also help.

Oddly enough, mild bladder inflammation can cause reflex pain in other parts of the body—when the bladder isn't even suspected. A 32-year-old woman suffered for years with a pain in the left shoulder which had been called "neuritis" by a number of doctors. She noticed she obtained some relief by drinking large quantities of spring water, but no connection was suspected between the shoulder pains and bladder irritation. A doctor cleansed her bladder with warm water (via catheter), and in four to five minutes the pain in her shoulder, which was very acute, entirely disappeared. After being convinced, she followed a cleansing diet for several days, and was completely relieved. That was four years ago, says the doctor, and the shoulder pain never returned. This doctor reports the next case.

A 52-year-old woman was confined to bed with an acute case of cystitis which had lasted over three weeks. As far back as she could remember there had been chronic irritation of the bladder, and all her life she had taken alkaline remedies to relieve the acid urine—until finally none of them gave her any relief. She was immediately put on a cleansing diet of water (in large quantity), and nothing else. Enemas were used, too. And as soon as her entire digestive system had cleaned out, all her bladder pains disappeared. After 10 days, raw milk every hour was substituted for water, and in a month she resumed a normal diet.

"There has been no return of the cystitis for more than eight years," says this doctor, "and neither treatments nor remedies have been used during that time." This relief came—after a lifetime of discomfort.

RAPID HEALING FOODS FOR KIDNEY, BLADDER AND URINARY PROBLEMS

Here is a complete list of rapid healing, rapid cleansing foods that have been used to relieve kidney, bladder and urinary problems. Starred items (*) refer to those foods which have proven especially useful. Foods extremely high in vitamin A, the factor known to help ward off stones and dissolve them, are marked (A):

*apple cider vinegar
*apples (A)
*asparagus (A)
bananas
barley water
beet juice, raw (A)
blackberries
blackeye pea hulls
blueberries
cabbage
cantaloupe
carrot juice (A)
cauliflower
celery
*cherry juice
*corn silk tea
*cucumber
*dandelion greens (A)
*garlic
gooseberries
*grapes
green peas (A)
honeydew
kale (A)

*kidney bean pod water
kohlrabi
*lemon juice
lettuce
mango (A)
melon
mustard greens (A)
nectarines (A)
*onions (boiled)
*parsley juice (A)
peaches
*pears
persimmons (A)
plums
pumpkin (A)
radish juice
sage tea
spinach (A)
squash (A)
strawberries
tomatoes (A)
turnip greens (A)
*water
*watercress (A)
*watermelon

Grapes have been known for centuries to have a cleansing effect on the entire body. Sanitaria in Europe have long prescribed the "grape cure." Grapes decrease acidity of urine, which explains why they have been used to relieve kidney, bladder and urinary problems. Their content of potassium tartrate helps wash out kidneys by increasing the flow of urine.

Watermelon has been known and used for centuries among European and other peoples as a mild stimulant to kidney action. Modern nutritional science has proved that an extract of watermelon seeds contains a substance called cucurbocitria, of value in dilating the large blood vessels and sometimes improving kidney function. Reportedly[1] watermelon is the best kidney and bladder flusher (diuretic), but if eaten in large gobs it won't work. It should be cut in little cubes, to hold in the mouth, one cube every three to five minutes. Do not eat or drink anything else that day. If watermelon is out of season, pears may do almost as well. These are also cubed into small portions and consumed every three to five minutes all day long. You will find yourself urinating more than you ever did before, says one doctor.

This doctor says that a spoonful of watercress-soaked water every few minutes during the day also acts as a powerful natural diuretic.[2] Alternating this with a day on watermelon has given relief and benefits to bladder cases when nothing else was able to help, he says. Merely soak a fresh supply of watercress in boiling water for an hour, or until cooked enough to drink, and take a spoonful of this every hour or so, for one full day, from early morning till sunset, not later. On the following day take a small cube of watermelon into your mouth every few minutes all day long, just for one day. The amount of fluid you will void during this period will amaze you, he says. It is a first-rate cleansing plan, and will clear up dribbling and frequent urination, he adds.

We are told that beet juice, in a way not yet clearly understood, clears debris out of human kidneys and is a kind of restorative and new lease on life. A single glassful of raw beet juice, freshly squeezed, is taken—1 teaspoonful every 10 min-

[1]*Doctor Morrison's Miracle Body Tune-Up for Rejuvenated Health*, by Marsh Morrison (Parker Publishing Company, Inc., West Nyack, N.Y.), 1973.

[2]*Doctor Morrison's Miracle Guide to Pain-Free Health and Longevity*, by Marsh Morrison (Parker Publishing Company, Inc., West Nyack, N.Y.), 1977.

utes—from morning till night. Nothing else that day. The urine may turn beet red (no harm). Do not drink in great quantities as this can cause upset.[3] Even kidney gravel and sulfa-formed crystals have been passed with this remedy.[4]

Tea derived from dandelion greens was used as an old-time herb remedy for kidney diseases and dropsy (edema). This vegetable is a kidney stimulant. It was also prescribed in ancient times to help treat stones. Today we know that dandelion greens are extremely high in vitamin A, the factor known to help ward off and dissolve stones and gravel.

Here are the most outstanding sources of vitamin A, in international units (I.U.) per 100 grams. Starred items have been used for kidney, bladder and urinary problems:

*asparagus	100,000
*dandelion greens	13,650
*carrots	12,000
*turnip greens	9,540
*spinach	9,420
*parsley	8,230
potato, sweet	7,700
*kale	7,540
collards	6,870
beet greens	6,700
*mustard greens	6,460
*mango	6,350
*squash, winter	4,950
*watercress	4,720
broccoli	3,500
*pumpkin	3,400
endives	3,000
chard	2,800
apricots	2,790
*persimmons	2,710
prunes, dried	1,890
papaya	1,750
*nectarines	1,650
*tomato	1,100
*apples	900
peas, baby	680
loquat	670

---

[3]Op. cit.

[4]*Doctor Morrison's Miracle Body Tune-Up for Rejuvenated Health,* Ibid.

Asparagus, in addition to being extremely high in vitamin A (which can dissolve stones), is rich in a food factor called asparagin, which acts as a gentle stimulant to kidney function, and is of particular value in cases of dropsy (edema). It is said that the juice of this vegetable helps the breaking up of oxalic acid crystals in the kidneys. A biochemist recommends cooked asparagus pureed, 4 tablespoons twice daily, morning and evening (diluted with water, if desired, and used as a cold or hot drink). It is harmless, he says, and has been known for 200 years to dissolve kidney stones.

He says that a woman's terminal kidney condition—inoperable—was cured with this method, after 30 operations for kidney stones failed (she attributes the cure entirely to asparagus); and a 68-year-old man's bladder tumor that failed to respond to any other treatment (including cobalt radiation) after 16 years, disappeared in three months with this asparagus treatment. Doctors confirmed that his bladder tumor was gone and his kidneys were normal.

Cherry juice can stop constant urination. One woman who was getting up from one to five times a night, and urinating every hour or so during the day, discovered that by drinking cherry juice, she scarcely knows she has a bladder—no more constant running to the bathroom. She can sleep a full seven hours without getting up. One teaspoon of concentrated cherry juice in a glass of water, several times a day, brings miraculous results, she says. Cherry juice can also relieve painful urinary infections better than antibiotics, in some cases.

Corn silk tea has a soothing effect on kidney, bladder and urinary problems, and can clear up pus, infection, burning or scalding urine, say users. Reportedly, it will also soothe inflammation of the urinary passages due to gravel or kidney stones, and regulate the flow of urine (whether too much or too little), in cases of bladder drip and incontinence—inability to hold urine—and urine retention or stoppage of urine. It seems to heal diseased areas of the kidney, bladder and urinary passages and flush out uric acid, toxins and other poisons.

Fresh cranberries can relieve bladder infections (they must be fresh, not canned). One woman found that by grinding them up, and sweetening them with honey, she can eat them at the first sign of trouble and ward off an attack. They work better than any medication she's taken in 40 years, and she's been free from bladder infections for a year, without drugs. She says they're delicious with plain yogurt and a satisfying bed-time snack.

Mr. L.B. says: "You may be interested in the following account of a very wonderful cure for a very infected kidney. In fact, it was so bad that the urine was almost white with pus. I am 85. At a local V.A. hospital, a Chinese doctor told me, 'Drink a glass of cranberry juice every day.' I have done this for over three years, and the latest x-rays and clear urine show that my kidneys are in excellent shape."

Garlic can relieve a persistent bladder infection (cystitis). Dice a little garlic, put it on a spoon and swallow it with water three times a day. This was tried by a woman who reported her cystitis disappeared in a few days.

Kidney bean pod water (the water in which the pods—not the beans—have been cooked) has brought remarkable permanent cures for kidney and bladder trouble. Heart patients suffering from dropsy or edema (excess fluid) have been completely relieved in two or three weeks, and stayed cured. It is a wonderful diuretic, causing large quantities of clear urine to be passed. Kidney blockage of long duration has been completely relieved, with this tea. Bleeding from any part of the urinary system quickly stopped, and did not return. Diseases of the bladder were cured! Stones and gravel were rapidly dissolved and did not return. Around 1900, the doctor who discovered it called it his "wonder cure." The pods must be fresh, the water no more than 24 hours old. Boil 2 ounces of pods in 3 quarts of water, slowly for four hours, filter through fine muslin, cool eight hours, strain again. Take one glassful every two hours. Old water causes diarrhea, and unfiltered water causes stomach upset. Otherwise, it is reported harmless and can be used indefinitely with excellent results.

Perhaps one of the most outstanding remedies is lemon juice. Although not high in vitamin A, lemon juice can dissolve kidney stones. Simply drink the juice of one or two lemons a day (mixed with water and sweetened to taste). Large kidney stones have been dissolved this way, and small ones immediately stop forming, says one doctor. Symptoms vanish at once, he says, adding that it was effective in about 50 percent of all cases of large kidney stones.

Parsley juice is valuable in removing poisons from the body, and is well-known for dissolving gravel and kidney stones. Culpepper wrote: "The seed is effectual to break the (kidney) stones and ease the pains and torments thereof..." Parsley tea has relieved pyelitis (inflammation of the kidneys), and other extremely painful kidney and bladder ailments. It has relieved prostate enlargement, with infection and pus, and complete stoppage of urine, avoiding surgery. Stir 1 teaspoonful of parsley leaves in a cup of hot water, cool, stir, strain and drink (1 cup, four times a day).

The *British Medical Journal* (Feb. 13, 1965), says that among those who drank large amounts of water (3-4 quarts daily), "clear signs of stone dissolution have appeared, results sometimes being spectacular."

For bladder problems, boiled water containing the pot liquor of a combination of pears, apples, peaches and plums has been recommended.[5] Take several spoonfuls when thirsty, or a spoonful every two hours, for three days, no other fluids allowed, only solids, says one doctor. After this, thirst may be quenched for the next three days only from melons, persimmons, tomatoes, apples, pears and peaches or nectarines. No soups or coffee or any other beverage for two weeks, he says.

To relieve burning urine, and painful urinary infections completely, in 24 hours, the following teas have been recommended: goldenseal, chaparral, lemon grass and Spanish eucalyptus. Any or all may be used, drinking about a quart an hour, and rotating the varieties to avoid boredom. Sweeten to taste.

---

[5]*Doctor Morrison's Miracle Body Tune-Up for Rejuvenated Health*, Ibid.

8

Rapid Healing Foods for Diabetes!

The pancreas is a tiny gland that produces insulin. Insulin is a hormone—secreted directly into the bloodstream—to enable sugar (from food) to leave the blood and pass into the cells for energy. When the pancreas is not working, excess sugar accumulates in the blood and eventually passes out of the body in the urine. The body becomes starved for energy. Appetite becomes enormous. But no matter how much is eaten, the sugar—the fuel—cannot be burned.

The sugar remains in the bloodstream, passes through the kidneys, and out of the body. The person develops many symptoms: weakness, dizziness, cold sweats, excessive thirst, frequent urination. When the sugar saturation of the blood reaches a certain point, it breaks down into poisons (ketones and acetones). The victim experiences shock, blackouts, coma and death.

This whole train of symptoms is called diabetes. Along the line, other organs besides the pancreas break down—like a domino effect—and the diabetic may develop kidney trouble, high blood pressure and heart failure.

ONCE A DIABETIC, ALWAYS A DIABETIC?

The pancreas, said Dr. William Howard Hay, like any other organ, can become intoxicated—poisoned—by the excesses of living. In his studies, the first time he used a cleansing diet to detoxify and cleanse a diabetic's body of poisons, all symptoms of diabetes, ravenous hunger, arid thirst, promptly disappeared. For three consecutive days he limited the patient's food to fresh unsweetened fruit juices and water only. This was followed by a diet of alkaline (non-acid forming) foods (these type foods are discussed in Chapter 1). "The hunger and thirst were never again uncontrollable, and the urinary sugar disappeared and soon the blood sugar was down to normal," he says.

"When we speak of cure," said Dr. Hay, "we can mean nothing less than a regeneration of this failing function ... Clean house and stop the causes of intoxication and you will have done all that bears any relation to recovery from this all too common generally misunderstood condition ..."

Dr. Hay continues: "Clean out the whole man and stop the intoxication that has overstrained this weak link. Then nothing can prevent return to health (in all but the most advanced cases)." If yours is a true case, he says, do not be discouraged, but also do not wait until you have reached an advanced stage and the pancreatic function is approaching nil. The ordinary case that has not used insulin is not at all difficult, he says, but if insulin has been used, degeneration progresses, and increasing doses of the drug are often needed.

THERE IS A CURE FOR DIABETES!

Medical doctors are not sure what causes diabetes, but they are sure of how to treat it. Once a diabetic, always a diabetic—that is the verdict in nearly all cases. In mild cases, a low-sugar diet is prescribed or an oral drug is given to help the body use sugar. In more severe cases, injections of insulin are given—and this is permanent, because it causes the pancreas to stop producing what little insulin it can.

Drugless doctors believe there is a cure for diabetes. They believe the pancreas can be built up again, and

that diabetes can be completely and permanently cured, in all but the most advanced cases—and even these can be helped. By removing the causes and correcting the eating habits, many cures have been achieved, they claim.

Life goes on a long time for the diabetic, because even if the pancreas is not working well, a little insulin is still usually produced. In addition, there are other glands and organs (like the adrenals) that secrete hormones similar to insulin to help use sugar. And there are many foods that contain insulin-like substances or help build up the pancreas.

AMAZING QUICK RECOVERIES!

In diabetes, we are told, a cleansing diet will remove the toxicity and waste infusions most speedily. After that, a well-balanced and properly combined starch-free diet must be adhered to, to re-establish metabolic balance. Good results have been achieved by going on a raw fruit and vegetable diet. Years before insulin, amazing permanent cures were achieved this way. As far back as 1926, an osteopathic drugless doctor stated:

"In spite of the seriousness of this disease, it is easily curable in the case of middle-aged patients ... The sugar in the urine will usually disappear after a few days, and will not again reappear, if the patient will rigidly follow instructions."

We owe much of our knowledge of the treatment of diabetes to the pioneering work of Henry Lindlahr, M.D., himself a victim of the disease. In the late 1880s, when men lived well and ate well, Henry Lindlahr (at 5'7") weighed over 250 pounds. He was proud of his wide girth (it was fashionable in those days—a sign of health and prosperity). To him, a brace of ducks was just a fine appetizer with which to begin a meal.

Then, at 31, just as he was ready to enjoy life, he developed advanced diabetes of the serious type—years before insulin. Treatment by all the best doctors and specialists failed. He was given up as hopeless and advised to settle his affairs. Death seemed inevitable, and he was prepared to accept it when, through the urging of a friend, he was persuaded to consult a famous drugless healer—Father Kneipp. This priest, who had turned healer in the little town of Woerishoffen, Bavaria, prescribed strict vegetarian diets, and a method of living that encompassed "a return to Nature." As Lindlahr's son, Victor (later to become a famed doctor and radio personality) recalled:

"Henry Lindlahr had absolutely no faith in the idea that a natural healer could help him. He went to Woerishoffen only to satisfy his friend. He had to wait 10 days for his appointment with Father Kneipp. In those 10 days, his eyes were opened to certain startling facts.

"He heard wonderous stories of the spectacular cures of this priest who leaned on Nature for his methods. He met patients who were healed of so-called incurable ailments—healed with diet, and natural methods. He found Woerishoffen to be a town of 15,000 people, grown in a few short years from a village of 500— with elaborate buildings erected to accommodate the patients of Father Kneipp.

"Finally, it was Henry Lindlahr's turn to see Father Kneipp. He received a shock when he stepped up for his few allotted minutes. The interview was short and to the point. Father Kneipp took a searching look at him, smelled his breath, and said bluntly: 'You are a pig! You eat too much! You are too fat! You have the sugar disease. You will take sitz baths and live on fruits and greens and vegetables. No bread, no cereals, no meats, no alcohol of any kind. See Sister Celeste.'

"Sister Celeste, one of Father Kneipp's assistants, gave him full details. He followed these instructions to the letter. His diet was purely vegetarian, very low in starches and with scarcely any fatty foods. Of course, today it is no miracle to us that a strict diet would rid a patient of excess sugar in the blood and its symptoms. But in those early days, a no-medicine treatment that really worked was startling!

"Springtime greeted a new Henry Lindlahr. His sugar was gone. He had lost over 40 pounds. His life had been saved. At 40, he made up his mind to study medicine and become a doctor, receiving his degree in 1904 ... At that time, unless there were some vaccine to use, serum to inject, operation to perform or medicine to give, the average doctor tended to be totally uninterested in prevention of disease ... However, Dr. Henry had been taught in a different school, that of experience.

"He knew beyond any doubt that he had developed diabetes because of his eating habits and his overweight...Because his sugar disease had been eradicated by a reform in his living habits, he realized that diabetes was not some accident ... And he was sure that if he had been warned or instructed as to the right way to live, he never would have violated Nature's laws..."

A STRANGE DISPENSARY

Dr. Lindlahr opened the first drugless clinic in the United States, the Lindlahr Sanitarium, in Chicago. At this clinic, drugs were expressly forbidden, even though Dr. Lindlahr and his staff (including his son) were doctors of medicine. "During the 20 years of his practice, it is doubtful if Dr. Henry wrote 100 prescriptions," his son recalled. Treating an average of 2,500 patients a year, many of them desperately sick men and women who came to him as a last resort, he actually practiced "medicine" without the use of medicines!

"Instead of the drugs and potions of his contemporaries, father gave his patients simple food and plant remedies. The Sanitarium medicine chest was in the pantry, the ice box and the cellar," his son recalls.

At the Lindlahr Sanitarium, the head cook was the chief pharmacist. The "wholesale drug supplier" was the food merchant from whom fresh vegetables were purchased. Dr. Lindlahr's "prescriptions" were his diet slips. He was not joking when he would say to a patient, "You need something for your nerves," and write on his note pad, "Buttermilk." Thus, a laxative might be mashed prunes; a tonic, pot liquors. To the informed nutritionist of today, these remedies of Dr. Lindlahr do not seem ridiculous.

FOODS AS MEDICINES

In 1908, Dr. Lindlahr wrote: "Many of our more common foods were once highly prized herbal medicines. Through hundreds of years they demonstrated their curative potencies which have never been lost except in the minds of men."

Cleansing diets were frequently used in the treatment of gall and kidney stone attacks, and to lower the blood pressure rapidly or to free a diabetic patient from excessive sugar. Said Dr. Lindlahr's son: "With all deference and respect to insulin, and the powerful depressants which have been developed to lower blood pressure temporarily, I doubt whether there are any more efficacious methods in use today of accomplishing these two results." Reduction in blood pressure was amazing—particularly in cases of impending apoplexy (stroke) where the pressure is dangerously high.

MANY AILMENTS VANISH

Dr. Lindlahr's son gives an example of how a leg ulcer, varicose vein, loose teeth, pyorrhea, aching joints, rheumatism and constipation—ailments which diabetics often suffer—were cured. One of his father's first patients was a Mr. W., a waiter with a grievous leg ulcer, a varicose vein and a bad case of scurvy. He recalls:

"Mr. W. was a man who drank alcoholic liquors too heartily and ate too much of the rich food he served. Pastries, fine meats and breadstuffs were his main food—he despised vegetables and fruits. His teeth were loose with pyorrhea, his joints aching with an established chronic rheumatism and his leg foul with the excrement of the ulcer. He had been constipated for nearly 20 years, and was addicted to laxatives...

- "When Mr. W. gave a history of 20 years of constipation, a little consideration of the fact that all the veins of the body must drain into the liver—an organ which is deeply involved in chronic constipation—gave a clue to why the veins of the legs were varicose.

- "When Mr. W. was put on a diet which freed him completely of constipation, a *cause* was removed. When Mr. W. was divorced from the use of laxatives, an abused, upset liver was given some surcease from its trials and troubles. Why, then, shouldn't the veins begin to drain more freely? Of course they should and they did.

- "When the circulation of blood through the veins of the leg was stimulated by cold water application twice a day and further encouraged and re-established by body massages, why shouldn't the varicose veins gradually recede? They should and they did.

- "With the fundamental causes of the varicose ulcer alleviated, with Mr. W. put on a diet exceedingly rich in healing vitamins and minerals and with the sloughing ulcer exposed to the healing, antiseptic rays of the sun, why shouldn't the ulcer heal? It did heal!

● "The same situation held for the condition of the gums. The disorder had a name, pyorrhea. Mr. W.'s teeth were loose and wobbly. Blood and pus would squirt from the gums if you touched them ... When Mr. W. recited the list of foods he ate, and told of his total dislike of vegetables, it was not difficult to diagnose it as scurvy (vitamin C deficiency)...

"Mr. W. was put on practically a fruit and vegetable diet, amplified by a daily quart of milk. He was forbidden to eat meats, breadstuffs and pastry with the exception of three slices of whole wheat bread a day. His leg was sunned for half an hour a day, gradually increased to two hours. He was given a general body massage three times a week and was ordered to allow cold running water to course over both legs for 15 minutes in the morning and for 15 minutes at night.

"Within six weeks, Mr. W.'s leg was healed. His teeth were firm and the gums, although receded, were healed..the fruit and vegetable diet had rid him of his constipation ... Not one of the many doctors Mr. W. had consulted had diagnosed his case as one of diet deficiency."

DIABETES CURED!

In another case Dr. Lindlahr's son recalls: "A patient came to us in the Spring of 1919 from Chattanooga, Tennessee. The wife of a well-to-do businessman, she was suffering primarily from diabetes but her case was complicated by high blood pressure and gallstones ... The prospect of coming to the Sanitarium had apparently induced Mrs. S. to have one last fling ... Mrs. S. had eaten three sumptuous meals aboard the train, and a typical farmer's breakfast at the station that morning before she took a cab to the Sanitarium ... By four o'clock that afternoon, there was a frantic call from her room. She had collapsed and was in a semi-coma. Apparently she had also undergone an aggravated gallstone attack, and her blood pressure ... was 260.

"Mrs. S. was, of course, put on a (cleansing diet)—she remained without solid food for 15 days. Then she was given our so-called LC (low-fat, low-carbohydrate) diet, consisting mainly of fruit and vegetables. By Christmas, she was absolutely cured, and I use the word cured knowing full well its implications...

"She returned to the Sanitarium the following three summers for checkups. Her blood pressure was never over 150, the gall bladder showed no pathological distortion and blood sugar stayed within a normal range ... her weight had been decreased from 204 or so pounds to about 160."

RAPID HEALING FOODS FOR DIABETES

In his book, *Health Secrets from Europe*, Dr. Paavo Airola says: "Even diabetics can try a (cleansing) raw juice diet, *but only under a doctor's control.* The carbohydrate content of juices is not high; besides, a certain amount of carbohydrate is good for diabetics. The leg ulcers of diabetics heal fast during juice therapy. Young diabetics should engage in sports; heavy physical work and exertion diminish the need for insulin.

"Juices for the treatment of diabetes are: green beans, nettles, cucumber, celery, watercress, lettuce, onions, garlic and citrus juices. Cucumber contains a hormone needed by the cells of the pancreas in order to produce insulin. The hormones contained in onions are also beneficial in diabetes.[1]

"Bean skin tea is considered by many biological doctors to be a natural substitute for insulin and extremely beneficial in diabetes. The skins of the pods of green beans are very rich in silic acid and certain hormonal substances which are closely related to insulin. One cup of bean skin tea is equal to at least 1 unit of insulin. The recommended dose: 1 cup of bean skin tea morning, noon and evening (Waerland system)."

Garlic has cleansed the blood of excess sugar. One method is to eat a combination of garlic, parsley and watercress daily. A British medical journal reported that garlic is as effective as tolbutamide in clearing the bloodstream of excess glucose.

---

[1]Onion and celery leaves are believed to contain insulin-like enzymes that burn off sugar.

Another method is to take a 5-gr. garlic capsule after each meal. This has lowered blood sugar in mild cases to the point where no drug was needed or prescribed. Reportedly, it normalizes low blood sugar as well.

Soybeans contain lecithin, an unsaturated fatty acid, which has apparently normalized many diabetics. One doctor reports curing diabetic patients with 6 tablespoons of soybean lecithin and 100 mg of vitamin E daily, over a period of weeks. He says patients reach the point where they can eat normally and no longer require insulin.

Honey can lower blood sugar, if used in place of regular sugar. That is because it contains levulose, a natural sugar which has the advantage of being absorbed so slowly that it does not have the shock effect of other sugars. It is Nature's answer to saccharine. A doctor reports giving honey to a diabetic patient for 10 days without an increase of sugar in the urine. With 4 teaspoons of honey daily, the sugar rate dropped. Another doctor used honey in the diet of 250 diabetic patients with success, and some people claim that in seemingly hopeless cases it has resulted in cures. The method used in one reported case was a diet of raw vegetables sweetened with honey and lime: spinach, lettuce, cabbage, carrots, fresh tomatoes and whole wheat bread. The person who used it said that a year later the doctors could not find a trace of sugar, and now, years later, he can eat anything on the table and do more work than any man his age (70).

Kidney bean pod tea has permanently cured diabetics. Around 1900, a doctor reported that diabetics who had taken this treatment 12 years previously—and stopped using it— stayed cured. Others whose sugar returned were able to find relief again by using it. Only the pods are used. They must be fresh. Boil 1 ounce in 4 quarts of water, slowly, for 4 hours, filter through fine muslin, cool 8 hours, strain again. Take one glassful every two hours. If the preparation is more than 24 hours old it causes diarrhea, and unfiltered water causes stomach upset. Otherwise, it is reportedly harmless. The length of time involved was three to four weeks, during which a strict diabetic diet was advised. More recently, one woman reported her sugar dropped from 326 to 128 in two weeks, and a kidney stone disappeared with this tea.

Blueberry tea can clear the blood of excess sugar, in mild cases. One woman used blueberry leaf tea two or three times a day for five months, on a diet of fruits, vegetables, lean meat and no sugar. She took the full range of vitamins and minerals, as well. At the end of this time her blood tested out perfectly normal.

Brewer's yeast can help the pancreas produce insulin, thus helping to prevent diabetes. In mild cases, it can be eaten for breakfast: have a sliced banana covered with wheat germ, ground sunflower seeds and brewer's yeast with milk. One woman who did this discovered that traces of sugar in her urine vanished.

Other foods that have been used to clear the blood of excess sugar include dandelion tea, and strawberries mixed together in equal portions with parsley and blueberry leaves (steep 1 teaspoonful in hot water, drink four times a day).

A recent news item stated: "Cantaloups, peanuts, grapefruit and whole grains may be more helpful to some diabetics than pills. They help nerve problems of burning and numbness of the feet, often associated with diabetes, according to Dr. Rex S. Clements, director of the Clinical Research Center at the University of Alabama Hospitals. Twenty percent of diabetics have these problems. The symptoms range from faint numbness or burning sensations in the feet to severe leg pain and loss of sensation. Cantaloups, peanuts, grapefruit and whole grains contain high concentrations of a drug called myoinositol, which relieves these symptoms. Diabetics can buy myoinositol in tablet form in health food stores, but Dr. Clements warns that they can poison the nerves. Complications can be avoided more easily with the dietary approach."

9

Rapid Healing Foods for the Thyroid!

Heart and circulatory problems of a serious nature may arise from thyroid trouble. The thyroid is a ductless gland that secretes its fluid directly into the bloodstream. It is located directly below the voice box. It regulates body metobolism—the rate at which you burn your food, and controls how much energy you have. It helps prepare waste matter for elimination. When it slows down, waste matter tends to pile up in the system, and you feel sluggish.

The two main causes of thyroid trouble, say drugless doctors, are lack of iodine, and the body's inability to keep itself clear of its own debris. Either one of these may cause thyroid trouble. For in many cases, it is not actual lack of iodine in food but rather a lack of power in the body to absorb it, due to a clogged, overstuffed system.

In almost every case, another factor will be noted besides iodine deficiency, and that is constipation. Reportedly, in most cases you will find a toxic state of the body induced by retention in the intestines. On a cleansing diet, or fast—not only is this

132

rubbish cleared out—but the body, forced to rely on its own reserves, will now use organic iodine which has been stored, but not completely assimilated. Thyroid function improves, symptoms vanish.

RAPID HEALING FOODS FOR THE THYROID

Rapid healing foods for the thyroid are those that feed it, and those that cleanse the entire system. The thyroid feeds on organic iodine contained in certain foods like garlic (the best source), onions, kelp, dulse, radishes, watercress, lemons, egg yolk and salt water fish such as haddock and cod. These foods are cleansing to the body and feed the thyroid gland. Iodine is not readily absorbed without vitamin E, but this is present in other cleansing foods, such as salads and green leafy vegetables.

When the thyroid lacks iodine, it may enlarge, causing a swelling at the base of the neck—called a goitre. By pressure on certain nerves and blood vessels leading to the eyes, or overproduction of fat in the sockets, it may cause the eyes to bulge. Symptoms of a sluggish thyroid are palpitation of the heart, extreme fatigue and severe headaches.

You are cold when other people are comfortable; your hands are clammy; your feet are so cold at night that you cannot get to sleep. You are mentally and physically sluggish. You gain weight easily, forever trying to reduce and forever staying too fat. And there may be blinding pressure headaches.

"CURE IS ALWAYS POSSIBLE"

There are many types of goitres, which only a doctor is qualified to diagnose and treat. However, one drugless doctor claimed that—regardless of the original cause—a cure is always possible through the use of a fruit fast. The thyroid is reduced in size, often the enlargement completely disappears, and the heart strain will be removed, he says.

This doctor reports the case of an 18-year-old girl whose neck was enlarged to about 18 inches, due to a goitre. She started fasting on the juice of one orange every two

hours, and continued this fast for a month. All signs of the enlarged thyroid entirely disappeared on the twentieth day.

To ensure a permanent cure, says this doctor, the orange juice fast was continued to the end of the month. Then she was put on the following diet:

Breakfast—1 egg.
  3 pieces brown, thin toast.
  Dish of stewed fruit.
Lunch— Choice of whatever desired of the following raw vegetables: spinach, asparagus, string beans, lettuce, celery, parsley, carrots, turnips, beets, parsnips.
Dinner— Small piece of broiled steak.
  2 cooked, nonstarchy vegetables.
  Salad of two or more nonstarchy vegetables.

This diet was continued for two weeks, and then other articles of food were added, until at the end of a month the patient was using almost any article of food desired. She was, however, advised to be cautious in the use of starches, and if they were used to use them only in small quantities, and always in proper combination with other food. "The patient has remained perfectly well for over eight years," said this doctor, "and about a year ago gave birth to a baby, without the strain of childbirth having any effect upon the thyroid. Her neck seems perfectly normal in every way, is well formed and there is no evidence of any enlargement of the thyroid gland."

BULGING BLOOD VESSEL, HEART AND THYROID HEALED

This doctor reported the following case. A disabled veteran, 24, was suffering from a bulging blood vessel (an aneurism of the thoracic aorta), valvular leakage of the heart and an enlarged and overactive thyroid (exophthalmic goitre with hyperthyroidism). He was receiving compensation from the government and was considered incurable. His systolic blood pressure was 180 mm, and his pulse was racing at 160 beats a minute, twice normal!

The government doctors had told him that he had about three months to live—a little longer if operated on, but

with no hope of permanent cure. He was immediately put on a cleansing diet by this drugless doctor. His improvement was so rapid from the very first, his blood pressure and pulse quickly returning to normal, that in less than a month, he started building his own house—clearing the land, and chopping wood himself!

Here is the diet that was used. He was told to drink a glass of orange juice three times daily, with a glass of water—and nothing else, no other food or drink. This was continued for 30 days. At the end of this fast, he was placed on a milk diet, taking 3 quarts daily, for a month. Then he was put on a well-balanced diet, being warned against too frequent use of starches, and by the end of three months, which was the time given him to live by the government doctors, he was apparently perfectly well.

"He has remained in good health ever since," said this doctor, "that is, for a period of about two years. A few days ago, I re-examined him and found no traces of the aneurism, the heart functioning perfectly in every way, blood pressure 120 mm systolic, and pulse 72. At the present time he is a perfect physical specimen of manhood, with no organic or functional defect."

10

Rapid Healing Foods
for Eyes, Ears, Nose
and Throat!

The eyes invariably become stronger during a cleansing diet, in some cases glasses may be discarded entirely, and eyesight is frequently restored to normal says one drugless doctor.

This doctor says that in one case, an entire family was able to stop wearing glasses (mother, father and four children). In another case, a young lady who had tried a cleansing diet for other reasons suddenly discovered her glasses were too strong, and eventually stopped wearing them entirely!

Hearing is definitely improved by a cleansing diet. Mucus and other gooey sludge that accumulates in the ear bones—making them rigid, and sometimes fused together—is dissolved by a cleansing diet. It is this mucus (catarrh) that is the acknowledged cause of over 90 percent of hearing problems. It is produced by many years of ingestion of too much refined starch foods, meats and other acid-producing foods.

HOW POISONS ARE ELIMINATED

During a cleansing diet, excess waste material in the mucus membranes of the nose and throat is among the first to be eliminated. As one drugless doctor points out, infections of the ear with the drainage of pus (as in ititis media) can be looked upon as an emergency waste removal from an overburdened body. This doctor notes that in a case of multiple sclerosis (the man had tried every other treatment and just got worse), after a two-week cleansing diet he almost cried when he realized he could move his toes for the first time in years—but even more amazing, a running ear, which had been bothering him since he was eight years old (for 26 years the body had been throwing off poisons in this manner), suddenly stopped as if by magic. This doctor says he has noticed the same thing in many similar cases.

A BLIND MAN SEES AGAIN!

With a cleansing diet, says one eye doctor, "Wonderful results have been obtained in conditions that seemed almost incurable. One case I recall: A gentleman went to a very reputable but orthodox medical institution to ascertain the reason for his failing vision. He was kept under observation for two months. During that time he lost his sight completely. He became very much discouraged with these great medical authorities, and decided that their reputation would not cure him ... This gentleman went to see a medical doctor who had practiced medicine for about 50 years, but who had decided that it was not scientific, and in the last few years had discarded his pill case and hypodermic needles.

"The good physician told the patient that the brain tumor, which had finally been the diagnosis of the other physicians who had suggested operation, was probably nothing more than congestion of the optic nerve as a result of a body loaded with poisons and toxins.

"The physician suggested a fast, and took him into his new health school, put him to bed, instructed one of his nurses to see that he was washed inside and out and given no food. On the twenty-first day of this treatment the patient began to see light and in 30 days not only did he have his sight, but his health was greatly improved, and after being taught what to eat he was again able to go back to his business.

"It is not my belief that it is safe for anyone and everyone to attempt a long fast without the aid of someone who thoroughly understands fasting, but the following plan of fasting can be followed by anyone of average intelligence without any danger.

"For instance, the fruit fast: Eat nothing but fresh fruits, absolutely nothing else but fresh raw fruits for three days. Then, fresh, raw vegetables, for three days, and be sure to wash the bowels out every day and drink water freely. Return then to a diet of two meals of fresh fruit and one meal of fresh vegetables each day for a period of two weeks. This has worked wonderfully and at the same time has permitted people to go about their regular work ... Another method that has been successful in a large number of cases is as follows: no food for three days, drink only water with a little lemon juice, no sweetening, washing the bowels out every day ... On the fourth day, one meal of fresh raw vegetables, chewed thoroughly; then gradually return to a normal diet (of foods that make you, see page 48)...

"Some patients have been such hearty eaters that their stomachs and intestines are dilated to several times their normal capacity; therefore, they cannot change suddenly from cooked foods to raw foods ... They must have a sufficient quantity of bulk, cooked foods to stimulate peristalsis. If you find, then, that raw foods cause you too much discomfort, you may have to add them gradually, increasing slowly the quantity of raw food and decreasing the quantity of cooked food. Moderation in all things (will) give the body a chance to unload, releasing the congestion, restoring normal structure and normal function."

AMAZING RELIEF FOR
EAR PROBLEMS

Hearing is one of the first body functions to improve on a cleansing diet. It grows clear and sharp. Barring certain ailments, like a punctured eardrum, and other conditions which only a doctor is qualified to diagnose and treat, many common hearing problems definitely improve on a cleansing diet. A doctor reports the following cases as proof:

"A retired doctor, 65, had been totally deaf for about 10 years. He suffered excess mucus in the nose and throat, and hoped I might be able to give him a diet that would relieve it. This was actually the cause of his deafness, which had forced him to retire. I explained the benefit of a (cleansing diet) ... and suggested that his hearing might be regained. Of course, he did not believe this, after eminent specialists had failed to help him.

"He started on an orange juice fast to rid his system of catarrh (mucus). During the fast he used only the juice of six oranges daily, one taken every two hours with a plentiful supply of water. After the tenth day, certain loud noises could be heard. His hearing continued to improve, and on the eighteenth day, he passed the test used for railway trainmen, and could hear a watch tick 18 inches from either ear. At the end of 25 days he was placed on the following 10-day diet:

"Three times a day soup made from the following vegetables: celery, asparagus, parsley, spinach. These were ground together in the raw state and then cooked for over an hour. After the cooking was completed he was allowed to add a small amount of butter and salt for seasoning. One or two bowls of this mixture were taken three times daily during the 10 days, and then the following diet was taken for several months:

Breakfast—Whites of 3 eggs.
　　　　　　3 or 4 pieces of thin, brown toast.
　　　　　　Dish of stewed fruit, selected from the following: figs, dates, raisins, apples.
Lunch—　A raw food meal, using a choice of the following: spinach, lettuce, string beans, carrots, turnips, asparagus, parsley, oyster plant, parsnips, beets.
Dinner—　Roast beef or beefsteak.
　　　　　　2 nonstarchy cooked vegetables.
　　　　　　Choice of the following salad vegetables: lettuce, tomatoes, cucumbers, celery.
　　　　　　No dessert.

"After several months of this diet the patient was allowed to make other changes in his diet, being careful to avoid inharmonious food mixtures, and cautioned to use a small amount of fats and starches. The cure was completed several years ago, and from time to time I have heard from the doctor, who has resumed practice, and has had no return of catarrhal symptoms or deafness.

"A four-year-old boy came to my office with his mother and his brother, aged two. The mother brought the two-year-old baby to be treated for enlarged tonsils, because she wished to avoid an operation, believing that a previous one was responsible for the older boy's deafness. I assured her that if the older child took the same diet treatment as the baby was to take to cure the enlarged tonsils, his hearing would be improved.

"And, in fact, the older boy followed the diet of the younger, and without any local treatments or any special advice, his hearing was completely restored. It has remained perfect ever since that time, which is now about a year ago (and the younger child's tonsils were reduced to normal size)."

MASTOIDITIS

Mastoiditis is an inflammation of the mastoid (a hollow part of one of the bones of the skull) behind the ear. In certain cases, this hollow space becomes filled with pus. This gathering of pus in the ear of a patient only takes place when the body contains an accumulation of wastes that need to be eliminated. This disease is quite common among children who have been fed an overabundance of sugars and starches. A slight earache, improperly treated, will often be the irritant that will cause the blood to deposit its poisons in the mastoid process. A surgical operation is usually advised to drain this pus from the cavity.

One drugless doctor says that, after successfully handling many serious cases of mastoiditis, he is convinced that it can almost always be cured by making use of the absorbing power of a cleansing diet. "No matter how young or old the patient may be who comes to me with an earache, he is immediately put upon (this cleansing diet) to ensure the immediate start of an absorption of pus, if any exists in the mastoid process," says this doctor. "This is always a safe procedure in any form of earache." He reports the following cases:

"A little girl, age two, had suffered from an earache for two days, and the eardrum was finally lanced by a doctor. The earache continued, and gradually localized behind the ear (mastoid). This doctor, an ear specialist, advised an operation. The mother asked me if this could be avoided. The baby was at once put upon a fast of water flavored with small amounts of orange juice. Three enemas daily were used, and hot applications administered to the upper part of the child's back. No treatment was given to the ear itself, because the eardrum had been ruptured, and I did not think it advisable to use either warm water or oil in the ear, although I did employ the radiations from an ultra-violet light lamp.

"On the second day, the discharge from the ear stopped entirely, and on the next day all symptoms of pain in the mastoid process completely disappeared. The baby was kept on the fast for a whole week, in order to make certain of a complete cure, and since that time has been using a diet such as I recommend as suitable for children. This cure was effected about a year and a half ago, and although the child had previously been subject to frequent earache, there has been no sign of any such symptoms since that time."

"A boy, 10, developed double mastoiditis; that is, inflammation of both mastoid processes. When I first examined him his temperature was 102 degrees, and both ears were discharging large amounts of pus. An immediate operation had been advised, but I did not think this necessary, and started the boy on a strict fast of water flavored with lemon juice. Both ears were treated with strong radiations from the ultra-violet light, and the fast was continued for 12 days.

"After the third day, all discharge in the ears ceased entirely, and the aching in the mastoid processes entirely disappeared the next day. At the end of the fast the patient was put upon a well-regulated diet, being careful to avoid an excess of starchy foods. Since that time, now about three years ago, he has had no return of the trouble."

EAR ABSCESSES DISAPPEAR

A professional singer, 35, had been greatly troubled with abscesses forming in his ears which had to be lanced from time to time, and his throat bothered him continually on account of enlarged tonsils. He was advised to take a glass of orange juice three times daily, with the addition of a glass of plain water, and to drink no other liquids or take any other food of any kind. One enema daily was taken. This patient was also grossly overweight, at 229 pounds. In the 15 days he remained on this diet, his weight was reduced 31 pounds. He was then placed on the following diet:

Breakfast—1 coddled egg.
2 pieces of thin, brown toast.
Dish of prunes.

Lunch—   Choice of one of the following raw fruits: peaches, pears, grapes, or 1 glass of orange juice.
One glass of water.

Dinner   Choice of one of the following: lean beef, mutton, chicken, turkey, rabbit or fish. Choice of one of the following cooked nonstarchy vegetables:

summer squash	celery
small green string beans	Swiss chard
spinach	asparagus
egg plant	oyster plant
beet tops	turnip tops
kale	mustard greens
cucumbers	chayotes
French artichokes	parsley
zucchini	lettuce

Choice of one of the following raw or salad vegetables:

watercress	celery
asparagus	parsley
cucumbers	lettuce
spinach	endive
tomatoes	

The doctor reports: "He is now following this diet regime, and is slowly reducing his weight until it becomes normal, which I think in his case will be about 175 pounds. The tonsils have been reduced to normal size, his voice is clearer than it has ever been and there has been no sign of any trouble in his ears since the date of the fast—nor will there be if he continues to live in accordance with the instructions given him."

ADENOIDS AND CHRONIC TONSILLITIS

Adenoids and tonsillitis can be quickly and entirely corrected with rapid cleansing foods, say drugless doctors. "The cure is quite simple," says one doctor. "These glands will return to their normal size and be clean and healthy. This is accomplished rapidly. After several days, the patient will be able to breathe freely with mouth closed. This may seem too good to be true, but it has worked in thousands of cases. You may expect remarkable results from a five-day cleansing diet, and better still, if continued for 10 days the adenoids will be reduced almost as rapidly as the tonsils with the same treatment. If you or your child happens to be suffering from any form of tonsil disease, try this treatment, and watch the miracle work."

Contrast this with the usual medical procedure, as outlined by Henry Lindlahr, some years ago:

"Many have heeded the siren call of the operating table and been sorry ever since. Here's why. After the tonsils have been removed, the work which they were doing must be carried on by other tissues, usually the adenoid tissues and nasal membranes. These, in turn, become hyperactive and inflamed, in many cases.

"Sometimes it happens that the adenoid tissues become affected before the tonsils. In that case, also, relief through the surgeon's knife is sought, and then the process is reversed: after the adenoids have been removed, the tonsils develop chronic catarrhal conditions.

"When both tonsils and adenoids have been removed, the nasal membranes may, in turn, become congested and swollen. Often the mucus elimination increases to an alarming degree, and frequently polypi and other growths make their appearance, or the turbinated bones soften and swell and obstruct the nasal passages, thus again making the patient a 'mouth breather.'

"When the nose takes up the work of missing tissues, the same mode of treatment is resorted to. The mucous membranes of the nose are now swabbed and sprayed with antiseptics and astringents, or 'burned' by cauterizers, electricity, etc. The polypi are cut out, and frequently parts of the turbinated bones as well, in order to open the air passages.

"Now, surely the patient must be cured. But, strange to say, new and more serious troubles arise. The sinuses or the throat areas are now affected by chronic catarrhal conditions and there is much annoyance from phlegm and mucus discharges which drop into the throat.

"When the drainage system of the nose and the nasopharyngeal cavities has been completely disorganized, the derangement may extend into the bronchi and the tissues of the lungs."

Now let's see how a drugless doctor might treat the same conditions. In one reported case, a child of two had difficulty breathing. His mouth was open with the tongue protruding most of the time. The child could not sleep more than an hour or so, at any time, day or night, because of the difficulty of breathing. A throat specialist said the child's tonsils were so enlarged as to almost entirely shut off air—and the nose was filled with adenoid growths. He advised an immediate operation. Before consenting, the parents brought the baby to an osteopathic drugless doctor, who immediately prescribed a cleansing diet, as follows:

Juice of 1 orange taken every three hours with half a glass of water (nothing else, no other food or drink).

Three enemas daily, each of a pint of warm water.

Two warm sponge baths daily.

This was started immediately, examination having been made about 1 p.m. "The change in the child's condition was so great during the remainder of the first day," says the doctor, "that he was able to sleep for 10 hours straight through that night. The tongue gradually drew back in the mouth during the next few days, and the tonsils were reduced in size, until at the end of seven days they seemed to be perfectly normal. From the very first night until the present time, the child has slept clear through the night. After the fast the following diet was prescribed:

Breakfast and lunch—The whites of 2 eggs cooked by heating them up with 2 tablespoonfuls of water in a dray pan over a slow fire.

2 pieces of thin, brown toast, moistened with hot water and seasoned with butter.

Small dish of stewed raisins.

Dinner—   Small piece of broiled steak.

Either cooked spinach or asparagus, and raw celery.

4 stewed prunes.

"This diet was continued for several weeks. The baby lost a little weight at first, because he was already overweight from the excess of starchy foods he had been using. Since then he has had other articles of food added to the diet ... At the present time the nose is entirely clear of any adenoid growths, the tonsils are normal in size, there is no protrusion of the tongue and breathing is entirely through the nose at night."

CURING SINUSITIS

Stuffed sinuses, with the usual congestion, pain, headache, pus and bloody mucus discharge, are a common problem. Years ago, William Howard Hay, M.D., who practiced medicine for 16 years and then gave up on drugs when his own health failed, devoting the rest of his life to drugless treatment, stated:

- "Sinusitis of every possible degree, treated in every possible environment, has responded to a detoxification and such dietary correction will again balance the body chemistry ...

- "The very same (method that) will cure sinus infection will cure it when applied to active cases of the most distressing types. It always has done so, and I see no reason to doubt that it always will when the laws of nature are in force.

- "Pan-sinusitis recovers as easily and usually as quickly as those limited to one sinus, for no matter how extensive the involvement, the discontinuance of the causes will result in nothing less than the cure ...

- "Neither does the climate or elevation offer a bar to complete recovery, for the condition comes directly from the foods eaten habitually, and these operate as cause or cure (regardless of climate) ...

- "Detoxification (a cleansing diet) will cure any case of sinusitis no matter how severe or how wide the involvement, and the cure is a matter of weeks ... without any change of climate, or environment or occupation, and without the expenditure of 1 cent for any type of treatment.

- "Again, I know this because it has always worked out just so, and I see no reason to doubt that it always will do so, for Nature is most kind in restoring us to normal if we will remove the former handicaps."

Dr. Hay explained: "Let us understand one thing clearly in the beginning, and this is that if you wish future ease (of sinus problems) never begin operations on this delicate region, for once begun there is no end to the damage done, and the end is far worse than simple, uncomplicated sinusitis ... The whole thing is so directly the result of wrong eating habits that it is easily within the control of the one afflicted ...

"When you have quit causing sinusitis you have already done the only thing at all constructive as regards its cure, and to attempt (to cure it any other way) is futile practice. The causes of sinusitis (and catarrh or mucus—are the same). No catarrh, no sinusitis, naturally ...

"If you will keep in mind the fact that internal filth or intoxication is the only cause of sinusitis I am sure the remedy for all degrees and types of the condition will suggest itself at once ... If now suffering from an acute and recent attack of sinusitis, stop everything and clean house first of all.

"On arising, or at any time when the stomach is empty, take 3 heaping tablespoonfuls of epsom or glauber salts ... to thoroughly flush out the body fluids as quickly as possible. This rapid extraction of body fluids will create thirst, and gratify this to the full with fresh unsweetened fruit juices, but no food, and no water except the distilled water that is found in this form in fresh fruit juices.

"If the trouble is quite recent this one purge may bring gratifying relief, but if the sinus is the seat of many previous similar inflammations it is quite likely that it will require several days of purging and fruit juice diet before there is a sensible relief. However long it requires do not make the mistake of eating anything further than the fruit juices till relief comes, after which there will be free discharge of mucus and pus ...

"To regenerate the body in any way is to stop all the causes of degeneration ... This means that we should eat more largely of the vital and base-forming groups of foods, for with few exceptions the devitalized foods are those productive of the greatest amount of acid ... When we have learned to eat only when hungry, of those foods we like best if they are not of the refined (pastry, candy, quick food) types; when we take these in compatible mixtures and when we are keeping the colon (clean) ... by daily flushing ... with 2 quarts of tepid or slightly cool water ... we shall not only recover readily and easily from any present sinus disease, but we shall at the very same time prevent the advent of future attacks..."[1]

---

[1]Many people believe that when they grow older, their sinus problem (or excess mucus) has disappeared. It has not disappeared, says Dr. Hay. It has entered the third stage—dryness. "Then the function of the mucous membrane is suspended. There is no sense of smell or taste, or these are very faint." This may explain why older folks often claim they have no appetite. It can be cured with this rapid cleansing plan, he says. The mucus will then pass through the fluid stage and be eliminated.

THE CAUSE AND CURE OF
HAY FEVER

There is no such thing as allergy, say the greatest advocates of the cleansing diet—drugless doctors who have cured thousands of seemingly hopeless cases. Allergy is not caused by an external substance (such as animal hair, pollen, strawberries, etc.). There is nothing wrong with those substances, for if there were, everyone would be allergic to them. One doctor claims:

- "The sufferer from hay fever can so change his body chemistry that he can bury his face in his former irritant no matter what this happens to be, without a single sneeze.

- "The victim of food allergy can then eat freely of this food without one slight discomfort, and with all the pleasure inherent in the eating of any enjoyable food.

- "It is not necessary to flee to the hills when hay fever season arrives, nor is it necessary to refrain from eating the foods we mostly enjoy ... Of the many hundreds of sufferers from hay fever who have (used this method), I know of no one today who is not free from the former irritations.

- "The same thing is true of asthmatics, for there is no such thing as an incurable case of either trouble."

The simplest explanation of hay fever and allergy is that they are *symptoms* of an overloading of toxins or poisons in the body, expressed through the mucous membranes of the eyes, nose and throat. They are actually drained at those points, just as poisons are drained from the intestines in diarrhea. The allergic substance is only a stimulus that makes the cup overflow (like the smell of food may nauseate you if you are ill). It is not itself the cause.

There is a specific reason why poisons accumulate in the system, faster than the body can eliminate them, which is the basic cause of practically all disease. It requires some explanation—and we will give the reason shortly—but if you are not looking for explanations, and only want quick results, accept the overloading of poisons as the simple reason for hay fever, and prove it to yourself.

Anyone can test this statement. Abstain from food—drink only fresh, pure (bottled) spring water—for a time and watch the nasal discharge and other symptoms of hay fever clear up. Thousands have recovered from hay fever by cleansing the system in this simple manner. As one drugless doctor points out:

- "Once the sufferer has been freed of his toxic load and the irritated state of the membranes of his eyes, nose and throat has been corrected, all symptoms of hay fever come to an end and they do not recur if he lives healthfully.

- "There is simply no need for anyone to go on, year after year, suffering with hay fever. Let the sufferer bear in mind that the pollens, the hair of animals and other substances to which he is sensitive or allergic, are normal elements in his environment and he will realize that his sensitivity to them must be due to something in himself."

- The healthy are not allergic, says this doctor, and it is mainly weakening habits—such as wrong foods and overeating—that are the cause of hay fever and allergies.

That is the simple explanation of hay fever and allergies, and the ridiculously easy way that you can cure them, permanently, in as little as 10 days to a month. It has worked in thousands and thousands of cases, say experts.

When cured with this method, an allergy sufferer can bathe in pollen without any ill effects, says one doctor. And the same is true of foods, cats or anything else. They will have no effect on you once you are cured with this method. The elimination of poisons in the respiratory tract results in a permanent clearing up of symptoms and the individual no longer suffers from allergies, he says.

If you wish more details—and another proven way to cure hay fever and allergies—here they are. We are a composite of what we eat daily, yearly and as a life habit. Allergy is not a condition affected so much by outside causes, but chiefly almost wholly, by what we eat and how we eat it. *When we eat too many acid-forming foods, we suffer.*

Many years ago, Dr. William Howard Hay explained it: *"A depletion of the normal alkaline reserve is behind every case of sensitization of every kind ... the creation of impossible amounts of acid end-products ... Starches and protein are highly acid* forming, as are all cereals, pastries, breads and sugars on the one hand, or meats, eggs, fish and cheese on the other ... When we consider that the average meal is composed of acid-forming material to the extent of 75 percent or more ... it is not hard to see why we continually accumulate these acid end-products."

Practically all ailments are caused by this lopsided eating of 75 percent acid-forming foods—say drugless doctors—when it should be just the other way around. Allergy sufferers and all other sufferers of ailments of almost every kind should eat 80 percent alkaline (acid-neutralizing) foods, says Dr. Hay. "To eat but a small amount of these acid-forming foods and a very much larger amount of the vegetables, the raw salads and fresh fruits, is to furnish both base-forming and acid-forming materials to the system in about the proportion in which they are continually lost through the body's processes.

"If the sufferer from allergies—whether food or pollen— would adopt this ratio of acid-forming (20 percent) to base-forming foods (80 percent) as a daily habit in eating, it would not be long until the former evidences of acid-alkali imbalance would disappear," says Dr. Hay. "*Always remember that every case of hay fever, asthma, eczema, psoriasis, food sensitivity or any evidence of allergy in any form, is never anything else but this same imbalance, meaning that the alkaline reserve has shrunk so low that the continual formation of acid end-products finds nothing to tie this excess or bind it into harmless compounds, and every evidence of allergy is entirely curable by a return to a normal acid-alkali ratio in eating.*

"Eat freely and largely of vegetables, salads, fruits; eat sparingly of meats, eggs, fish, breads, cereals, pastries, sugars, and you will build up an alkaline reserve that *will make the appearance of allergy impossible*," says Dr. Hay, and you can prove this to yourself right now, he says, to your complete satisfaction. Start a few months before the allergy season and sail through it.

SERIOUS CASES OF HAY FEVER CURED

We are told of a woman, 33, so weak from hay fever and allergies she could not walk more than a few steps at a time. A drugless practitioner showed her how to use the cleansing diet. For more than 40 years she has had no recurrence of hay fever—and has lived all this time in southern climates where the air is filled with pollen almost all year. At 73, she is busy, active, and in good health.

A doctor reported the following case: "A married woman, 40, had suffered from catarrh (excess mucus) all her life, with hay fever during the months of May, June and July each year. She came to my office at the start of one of her hay fever attacks three years ago, in May. Her eyes and nose were red, and she was forced to wipe them almost constantly. She sneezed so violently and often that it was impossible for her to go out much in public.

"A fast was started, using only plain water, and drinking a glass every half hour during the entire day. No fruit juices were used in this fast ... although the fruit fast will sometimes have beneficial results, my experience is that *every case responds to the plain water fast.*

"The fast was continued for nine days. On the second day the sneezing stopped, and at about the sixth day all signs of hay fever had disappeared. The patient received daily ultra-violet light (from a quartz mercury vapor lamp) which helped. *I suggested that the patient drive out into the country and walk through the hay fields, in order to convince her that the cure had been made through a cleansing of the bloodstream*, and that if she remained in a condition free from catarrh, she need never fear any slight irritation which might be produced by the smell of hay or the pollen of plants. *She has remained well, and without a sign of hay fever, during three seasons, and seems to be completely cured."*

"As I am writing this in the month of August," said this doctor, "I feel it might be helpful to my readers to report a case recently called to my attention of a woman, 34, who used (a cleansing diet) to cure a stomach ulcer, and found—to her surprise—when the hay fever season rolled around, she had no sign of it (she had been suffering every year, since childhood). She was an actress, and her hay fever had been so bad that many times she had to cancel theatrical engagements, simply because she could not go through a performance without sneezing constantly. Now she was cured."

RAPID HEALING FOODS FOR
EYES, EARS, NOSE, THROAT

Glaucoma has been rapidly relieved by drinking the water in which carrots have been boiled. In one advanced case, the man could only see shadows. He began eating three carrots a day, boiled in a quart of water, and drank the water, without seasoning. In nine days, he began to regain sight. After two months, he can see shapes and colors, and identified a friend's Volkswagen parked across the street.

Soybean lecithin can improve eyesight by cleaning out veins and arteries and improving circulation. A man with blurry eyesight reported that by taking 3 tablespoons of soybean lecithin a day, in two weeks his vision cleared up. Soybeans help break up fat, and placing sufferers on a low-fat diet is one means eye doctors have of halting deterioration of the macula lutea in the center of the eye and saving sight.

Foods that can help correct cataract include the tops of vegetables, turnip greens, parsley, mustard greens, dandelion greens, watercress, beet greens, common beans, milk and eggs. Liver and sunflower seed meal were used by a 90-year-old woman going blind from cataracts (dimming vision, red weepy eyes and a noticeable film). At 94 her cataracts are gone and her mental and physical health improved tremendously. Brewer's yeast, liver and soybean lecithin were used by another man to dissolve his cataracts and avoid surgery. Olive oil, applied to the eyes and eyelids, was used by a man to get rid of a very painful film over his eyes. He claimed that after two or three applications, his sight was entirely restored. Goldenseal tincture or fluid extract, applied externally to the eye in a dilution of 2 drops in an eye bath will heal a corneal ulcer if used three times daily, say researchers.

Sunflower seeds have been found to relieve farsightedness, eyestrain, ache and pain and extreme light sensitivity, such as the bright reflection from snow or the glare of automobile headlights and TV screens. One man, a Mr. H.B., says: "Sunflower seeds have done a lot of good for me. I needed reading glasses since I was 45 years old, am 65 now, have eaten the seeds for about two years or more and can read a lot now without glasses." Another man, Mr. F.N., says: "I brought my eyesight back with sunflower seeds, 3 teaspoonfuls of the kernels a day. Everything was a blur, but now I can read without glasses. Even my hair is getting life and luster back into it."

The enthusiastic reports about sunflower seeds continue. Mr. S.G. says: "Having had severe eye trouble for many years, I decided to try (sunflower) seeds. I ate a good-sized handful each day, and in about two weeks I noticed a definite and almost unbelievable change. The strain, ache and pain almost completely disappeared and I could work the entire day without being conscious of any trouble. An eye specialist (one of the best) after an examination stated that my eyes had improved and he prescribed weaker lenses."

"The very first time I ate sunflower seeds I felt results," says Mr. J.S. "I knew then and there that sunflower seeds were good for me and something my eyes needed. And the more I have eaten, the better they get. The results are immediate and at the same time lasting." Mrs. O.B. writes: "I am 66 years old and have always worn glasses. I have unusually far vision, so objects near were hard to distinguish ... I have never taken vitamins in any amount. I use about half a cup of sunflower seeds a day. I eat while ironing, walking, while on the bus or while reading or listening to the radio. I can at times thread a needle and sew without the aid of glasses. I often go all day without glasses, which I have not been able to do for many years ... I feel the seeds are really helping me to restore my eyesight."

Soybean lecithin can improve hearing. One man complained of deafness and a ringing noise in his ear. When he began to use lots of soybean lecithin every day, suddenly the ringing stopped and his hearing cleared. He is so happy that he plans to keep using this cleansing food that improves circulation and cleans out fat-encrusted veins and and arteries, causing sudden improvement in many cases.

Garlic oil can relieve earaches. One woman reports: "I have seen it work wonders within 10 to 15 minutes of puncturing a garlic oil capsule, pouring it into the ear and stopping it with a little cotton. I have told friends and relatives about how the pain stops soon after, and they all swear by it. My sister had an inner ear infection and cried all through the night with pain. She called me at 4:00 a.m. in tears. Her husband came and got some oil and the pain was relieved in 15 minutes." Onion juice can relieve bad hearing and ringing ears. One man says: "My ears would ring so much and my hearing was very cloudy. Three years ago I read, 'It is said that a drop of onion juice in the ear is good for hearing.' I tried it with wonderful results. Start about three times a week and as your condition improves you may cut down. I now use it about every week or 10 days and maintain good results."

Violet leaf tea can relieve throat pain, when used as a gargle. It is so powerful that—while not a cure—it has been used to relieve the horrible pains of throat cancer. Sufferers have said that only this tea, used as a drink, mouthwash or gargle, relieved their agony.

Garlic can cure a cold. A doctor reported that if one puts a piece of garlic in the mouth, at the onset of a cold, on both sides between cheek and teeth, the cold will disappear within a few hours or, at most, within a day. In 71 cases, clogged and running noses completely cleared up in 13 to 20 minutes with garlic. Coughing was relieved. It can relieve a sore throat in minutes, and completely relieve a sinus headache. It works faster than vitamin C, and gives permanent, not just temporary relief. Garlic also has a curative effect on chronic diseases of upper respiratory organs—absorbing poisons—and this is true for chronic inflammation of the tonsils, salivary glands, and neighboring lymph glands, empyema of the maxillary sinus, severe pharyngitis and laryngitis, says one doctor, adding that it "makes loose teeth take root again, removes tartar," and has a curative effect on eye catarrh and inflammation of the lacrymal (tear) duct, can relieve an ear ache (just wrap the plant in gauze and place it in the outer ear canal), and can relieve a headache, dilating the veins and arteries to relieve congestion (just squeeze some garlic juice into a teaspoon of honey). It is nature's aspirin.

Cod-liver oil can relieve sinus problems. Its high vitamin A has a healing effect on the mucous membranes of the nose and throat. Mrs. W.L. says: "I would like to tell you of the good results I have had with cod-liver oil. For 11 years I suffered from congested, infected, painful sinuses. Doctors usually prescribed antibiotics and anti-histamines that did not give satisfactory relief. The condition worsened, producing blood in the mucus. Alarmed, I consulted a specialist. But all he could do was write out two standard prescriptions. Then I remembered my grandmother had given me cod-liver oil as a child. I thought it might help the mucous membrane of my sinuses and throat. I started taking 1 tablespoon of cod-liver oil a day. In four weeks the bleeding stopped. Now I take 1 tablet every other day. This has saved me time and money: fewer sick days from work, lower doctor bills, less medicine."

Dolomite may relieve a condition known as "black tongue." Mr. D.O. says: "For about seven years I was bothered with 'black tongue.' My tongue would turn altogether black for a few weeks, then clear up for a few weeks (although it was coated, never pink). I consulted at least a dozen doctors about this and none of them could prescribe a remedy. Finally, I purchased some dolomite and took 6 tablets a day—2 after each meal. Within a week my tongue became a beautiful pink. That was about six months ago. I am still taking the dolomite and have had no further trouble."

Epsom salt can relieve excruciating tooth and gum pain instantly. One woman reports that after having a tooth pulled, that side of her mouth hurt so badly she was almost hysterical. She quickly gargled with a mixture of epsom salt and hot water. It worked like magic, and whenever the pain came back, the same simple remedy banished it. By the end of the day all pain was completely gone.

Honey can relieve hay fever. In Vermont, hay fever victims chew on honeycombs before, during, and after the hay fever season, and take honey mixed with apple-cider vinegar three or four times a day. Chewing honeycombs keeps the nasal passages open and acts as a sedative. For 25 years, one man suffered from hay fever every June. Then he tried chewing on a teaspoonful of honeycomb during a severe attack. The hay fever vanished in seconds, and each time it recurred, the same simple remedy banished it. Others report the same amazing relief from ordinary honey—claiming they no longer need allergy shots. Reportedly, fall honey is best.

Comfrey can relieve hay fever. One man simply eats two comfrey leaves a day. This has completely controlled his hay fever. He has recommended this to others, with the same results—a complete end to hay fever so long as comfrey is eaten throughout the season. After about a week, symptoms of drippy nose, itchy eyes, etc., vanish. Comfrey tea can relieve asthmatic or allergy night coughs. About ¼ to ½ cup of strong comfrey tea with a teaspoon of honey can end a coughing spell and bring restful sleep. Users claim it seems like a miracle. Relief seems permanent, with no side effects.

Garlic is an effective remedy for virus and other infections. Six cloves are chopped and added to green salad, or crushed and blended with butter and spread on bread or toast. In addition, one drinks a glassful of hot water in which has been stirred 4 tablespoons of cider vinegar and 2 tablespoons of honey. A man plagued with respiratory allergy problems tried garlic oil (10 drops daily), and says: "The results are like a new religious experience. I was one who felt the results in seven days. The comfort and ease I feel now is beyond description." Garlic can also relieve sneezing. One man had been sneezing for four days. Nothing doctors gave him stopped the spasms until he was given lots of garlic. Almost immediately, the sneezing stopped. In another case, a woman who'd been sneezing for six days got the same amazing relief with garlic.

Rose petal tea can relieve hay fever. Symptoms of sore and irritated eyes are relieved by steeping a few rose petals in a cup of hot water. This is carefully filtered, and the liquid applied to each eye four or five times a day. Estivin, a widely used eyedrop for relief of hay fever, is a "processed infusion of rose petals."

Orange peel can relieve allergies. One woman says: "I have found orange peel to be the best anti-histamine I have ever tried. I have been a victim of allergies all my life." She saves the peels, cuts them in small strips and soaks them in apple cider vinegar for a few hours. She drains them, puts them in a pan with honey and cooks to just before the candy stage. "I put them in the refrigerator and eat as I need them (like just before bed). No more stuffiness and clogged air passages to keep waking me from sleep." Tangerine peel can relieve a runny nose. Says one man: "It works! Stops running nose within 5 to 10 minutes." He just chews a small dry piece and swallows it.

QUICK RUNDOWN OF FOODS
THAT HAVE BEEN USED
IN TREATING SPECIFIC AILMENTS

In the following lists, please note that foods rich in vitamin A marked (A) are especially healing to the mucous membrane lining of all organs, such as the eyes, nose and throat. They keep this membrane moist, healthy and resistant to germs and infections. For a more complete list of foods rich in vitamin A, see pages 118-119.

Eyesight

acerola cherries
artichokes
beet green (A)
brewer's yeast
carrots
   (glaucoma, A)
carrot tops (A)
corn
dandelion greens
   (A)
eggs
goldenseal
   (corneal ulcers)
liver
milk
mustard greens
   (A)
olive oil
parsley (A)
potato (raw,
   crushed, as
   poultice for
   sore eyes)
soybean lecithin
squash (A)
strawberry
   (crushed,
   poultice for
   sore eyes)
sunflower seeds

turnip greens (A)
watercress (A)

Cataract

beet greens (A)
brewer's yeast
carrot tops (A)
dandelion greens
   (A)
eggs
liver
mustard greens
   (A)
parsley (A)
soybean lecithin
sunflower seeds
turnip greens (A)
watercress (A)

*Cold, Flu, Virus,
   Coughs and
   Fevers*

artichokes
beet greens (A)
carrots (A)
elderberry (A)
garlic
grapefruit[2]
green peppers (A)
green snap beans

leeks
lemon juice
onions
oranges
parsley (A)
scallions
tangerines
tomato (A)

Hearing

garlic oil
   (earaches)
onion juice
   (ringing)
soybean leci-
   thin (oto-
   sclerosis)

*Hay Fever
and
Allergies*

comfrey (leaf
   or tea)
garlic
honey
honeycomb
orange peel
rose petal
tea
tangerine
   peel

---

[2]Reportedly, many physicians recommend the grapefruit cure for colds, flu and fevers: no solids whatsoever, plenty of water and from 5 to 15 grapefruits a day.

11

Rapid Healing Foods for the Nerves!

Headache is one of the first symptoms of poisons in the system—and one of the first to disappear quickly and permanently, with rapid cleansing foods. Practically *all* of the many *kinds* of headaches are mere manifestations of this one basic cause.[1] Clear the system of poisons, and headaches will vanish, whether they arise from liver, gall bladder or kidney trouble, anemia, high blood pressure, low blood pressure, heart, vein or artery problems, eye, ear and nose problems, male or female problems or constipation, say drugless doctors.

As William Howard Hay, M.D. explained it, "In migraine, or common sick headache, toxins are developed up to the point of tolerance, the highest point at which the body can function, and here develops a crisis (a headache) that is the characteristic effort of the body to find relief from the increasing intoxication.

"The entire object of the attack is to unload these toxins and return to a less toxic state; hence (in migraine), the sickness, the

---

[1]Headaches due to sunstroke, or vertebra displacement, are among the few exceptions.

157

vomiting, the repugnance for foods of all kinds ... To be sure this does not return the body to a point that could be called normal, but only to a point that allows of function about as usual, and every sufferer from migraine knows how well the body feels for a time after each attack."

REMOVE THE CAUSE
AND CURE THE HEADACHE

Headaches are not *caused* by liver trouble, constipation or any of the other ailments cited above—for these ailments are only *symptoms* of poisoning in various parts of the body, and symptoms do not cause each other. Drugless doctors say:

The cause of headaches is poisons in the system. Remove the poisons and the headaches disappear. The poisons are nearly always poor food combinations. Two good foods—eaten together—can be a deadly mixture, whereas alone or with other like foods they are harmless.

Long-standing (20-year) sufferers of migraine and other headaches have found complete and permanent relief, practically overnight, with this simple method. As Dr. Hay explains it: "It is a simple thing to empty the colon daily by means of a 2-quart cool enema of plain water, which does no harm of any kind ... this measure will actually cure a very large percentage of cases, I think it safe to say 50 percent or more of them.

"Then, to complete the guarantee of permanent relief, separate the foods into compatible groups, and you will soon find yourself eating about the same foods as usual but without headaches of any kind." Dr. Hay further explains this food combining method as follows:

1. At one meal, eat only carbohydrate foods, including sweets and starches. Eat vegetables, salads and sweet fruits or sweet desserts, but no acid fruits, no acid dressing on salads, and no meat. Sweetened coffee, if desired.

2. At a different meal, eat only meats or other concentrated proteins, vegetables (avoid starchy vegetables like potato), raw salads, acid fruits (but not sweet fruits). Dessert: only fruit or gelatin. Unsweetened coffee only, if desired.

3. Do not use milk with meal #1 (starches, sweets) *or* with meal #2 (protein, acid fruits). Use milk only with an all vegetable meal.

In other words, combine in one digestive task only those foods that have similar digestive requirements. Do not eat together those foods that cannot possibly digest together in the same stomach at the same time. Only eat when hungry, and avoid refined or processed foods.

Starchy or sweet foods include all cereals, breads, starchy roots, such as potato or winter squash, as well as all kinds of sugars. Chew them well, for a large part of their digestion occurs in the mouth. And do not take an acid food (a citrus fruit, for example) in your mouth at the same time, as this will neutralize your saliva.

The concentrated protein foods include meats of all kinds, game, fish, cheese, eggs. These may be eaten with any acid food, such as citrus fruit. Digestion of these occurs only in a positively acid medium—that is, the stomach.

Carbohydrates (starches and sweets) require an alkaline condition in the stomach for complete digestion. Proteins (meat, egg, fish, cheese) require an acid medium to digest fully. *When you take both into your stomach at the same time, you are asking your stomach to be both acid and alkaline, which is impossible.* As a result, the carbohydrates never get fully digested. Neither do the proteins. When these undigested foods reach your intestines, they ferment, creating all sorts of noxious gases and poisons that are the basis of many ailments.

HEADACHE RELIEVED
AFTER 68 YEARS!

Dr. Hay recalls: "A few years ago an elderly lady of 83 asked to see me before a lecture, saying she had something to tell me that she thought might interest me. She reported that, three months before, her son had come to me for indigestion, and I had prescribed for him, and she thought to make it easier for him by following the same diet. Of course it was not a special diet, for indigestion needs nothing except a correction of the usual mistakes.

"She reported that since she was 15 years of age she had
suffered every day of her life with headaches; not the
familiar migraine, which is always periodic, but with a
continuous headache. Keep in mind that she was then
83 and had suffered every day since she was 15. She
reported that since she had been eating as I had directed ... all her headaches had left her ... within the
first week.

"All this means that her headaches were toxic, as what
headache is not, and that these toxins were created by her daily
intake at the table. Every day of her life she ate her foods in
incompatible combination, apparently, for she was still eating
the same foods as formerly, but was separating them into
compatible groups, having made absolutely no other changes in
her eating habits ...

"Except for the great length of time these headaches had
persisted, this same evidence could be adduced in many hundreds of cases of shorter duration reporting that, after thoroughly cleaning house and separating their foods into
compatible groups, not one headache had developed ... If the
colon is (flushed), it is safe to say that half the customary
headaches would disappear immediately."

NERVE AILMENTS CURED

Seemingly hopeless nerve ailments have been cured with a
rapid cleansing diet. And I say seemingly hopeless because it is
a well-known fact that nerve tissue cannot heal once destroyed.
Yet there are many reported cures, in documented cases. This
may be due to the fact that many nerve ailments seem completely curable in the early stages, say drugless doctors. And
results approaching cure have been obtained even in advanced
cases. In addition, deep states of internal toxemia (excess waste
material in the body) often simulate (or act like) nerve degeneration. Dr. Hay says:

"Peripheral neuritis is, without doubt, primarily a toxic
state in which degeneration of the nerve terminals develops only
after long-continued irritation of these terminals by enormous
accumulations of toxic materials. Such cases are possible of
recovery at any time before actual degeneration sets in ... Many

such cases have cleared up completely by detoxication and dietary correction (even though they had been diagnosed as degenerative)...

"Tingling of the toes and fingers, gradual loss of sensation in the terminal nerves, numb sensations, arms and legs 'going to sleep' continually, gradual loss of motion and power in the extremities—these are the usual symptoms of peripheral neuritis. If such symptoms are present do not accept the diagnosis of a degenerative change until you have cleaned house thoroughly and arrested the manufacture of toxins, for you may be agreeably surprised to find the illness clearing up when you have lowered the toxic level in the tissues."

SHAKING PALSY DISAPPEARS

Paralysis agitans, also known as shaking palsy and Parkinson's disease, develops late in life, usually after the age of 40. The shaking occurs more when the victim is sitting still, and less when active, but is certainly enough to make many tasks (like writing) difficult. It starts with a fine tremor and a feeling of weakness, usually in one hand or arm. In the beginning, the shaking can be controlled by the will, but as it progresses this is not possible. In advanced stages, there is often dullness of mind, drooling, a tendency to go forward (the so-called propulsion walk) and restlessness of the fingers. The tongue and chin may become tremulous, the shaking violent at times. It has no known cause, and medical doctors say there is no remedy for shaking palsy.

> Yet drugless doctors say this ailment may be completely curable in the early stage. And results approaching cure have been obtained even in advanced cases. In practically every case (with a cleansing diet or fast), patients make sufficient progress to become useful again, with but a slight tremor, and excellent results may be obtained in the great majority of cases in a comparatively short time, says one drugless doctor.

Drugless treatment consists of a fast (or cleansing diet), during which all shaking usually stops. When eating is resumed, the shaking resumes, but is less severe. After a time, a second fast is begun, with the same results, the shaking being even less when eating is resumed. A third fast is often enough to result in a complete cessation of tremors. In some cases a fourth or fifth fast is required. Complete recovery, where possible, is a matter of months or longer.

Eating between fasts is limited, and confined largely to fresh fruits and fresh (preferably uncooked) vegetables, with nuts or an unprocessed, mild cheese for protein. Bread, meat, salt, condiments, coffee, tea and cocoa are avoided completely, as are smoking and alcohol. Plenty of rest and sleep are recommended. Sunbaths are reportedly helpful, but not in excess. Light exercise (movements requiring skill rather than strength) is recommended when eating is resumed.

Reported cases:

- A woman, 40, had suffered with Parkinson's disease for six years. She had received the finest medical care available, with no results. She grew progressively worse. Then she went to a drugless clinic, where she was put to bed and placed on a fast (or cleansing diet). She soon regained control of her limbs. After a month, normal eating was resumed, but the tremor reappeared. A second and third fast were used. Each time, the tremor grew less and disappeared entirely after the third fast, with no recurrence. For more than 10 years, she has remained well, leads a busy, active life and enjoys better-than-average health. (Total treatment was nine months.)

- A woman with Wilson's disease (which so greatly resembles Parkinson's that it is difficult to tell them apart), with enlargement and hardening of the liver, used cleansing diets or fasts over a period of three months—under the care of a drugless doctor. She had been unable to write for many years, due to violent shaking. In two weeks, she was able to write letters, and her hands were as steady as a normal person's. She was satisfied with her results, and felt no further treatment necessary.

Patients often live for as many as 20 or more years after Parkinson's symptoms begin. Its cause is said to be "entirely unknown." Nervous tension and exhaustion after some trying experiences seem to have something to do with it. Overindulgence in work or play (especially sex) seem to be factors.

Overeating or anything that leads to nervous fatigue may bring it on.

MULTIPLE SCLEROSIS

Multiple sclerosis results in hardening (sclerosis) of the nerves in the brain or spinal cord. However, not all the nerves are affected. It occurs in sporadic patches. The nerve covering breaks down and nerve cells and fibers fuse together. This is gradual and starts only as an inflammation. Because not all the nerves are affected, some work energetically, some weakly, some not at all. No two cases are alike. The hardening occurs in different places in different people, and not at the same rate of speed. Symptoms include weakness, strong jerky movements, lack of coordination, especially in the arms, hallucinations, impaired speech, involuntary rapid eye movement. Beginning symptoms come and go. These include loss of vision in one eye, double vision, tingling or numbness, weakness in the legs, difficulty walking, incontinence. They are mild and may come and go for years in the beginning. *This indicates that something can be done*, say drugless doctors, while medical doctors say it is incurable.

One drugless doctor claims there is a possibility of recovery in thousands of cases now regarded as hopelessly incurable. "I have been able to return some of these, even in helpless conditions," he says, and he feels early cases may be completely curable.

"It is in the initial stage that full recovery is or should be possible," he says. Drugless treatment consists of a series of fasts (or cleansing diets). The first one, he says, "brings about remarkable improvement in the general health of the individual with considerable increase in his control and use of his limbs, often enabling the bed-ridden patient to get up and walk." This is followed by a carefully planned diet, regular exercise and sunbaths. A second fast adds to his control and use of his limbs. Then a third fast. Between fasts, there is rest in bed, light exercise requiring skill rather than strength, and a diet of fresh fruits and vegetables, with only moderate amounts of fat, sugar, starch or protein. This doctor prefers vegetable proteins—nuts and sunflower seeds are especially good, he says. (See page 167.)

EPILEPSY

Medical doctors state that epilepsy can be controlled but not cured. We are told, however, by one drugless doctor (an osteopath) that "a cure may be looked for if the strictest regime is followed faithfully and long enough to cleanse the system entirely from the virulent toxemia which is responsible for the disorder."

Often after several days, the violent and repeated spells will stop entirely, and no more will occur if the cleansing diet is continued, followed afterwards by correct foods, he says, adding that attacks will be further and further apart, until they cease altogether.

"After the cure," he says, "the patient must be content not to overeat, and the bowels must be kept freely open ... For some time after the cure seems certain, two enemas daily should be taken, with 1 quart of warm water each time, in the knee-chest position ... Sometimes the seizures will occur more often than usual at the start of the fast, and this may be regarded as a good sign that the poisons are being stirred up by the systemic housecleaning."

This doctor reports the case of a man, 32, who had been experiencing epileptic seizures since he was 24. "The patient was put on a fast of grapefruit every two hours during the day, combined with a glass of water. The first night of this fast 4 ounces of olive oil and 4 ounces of grapefruit juice were taken together just before retiring, in order to stimulate the action of the liver and gall bladder. This fast was taken for 14 days. No attack occurred during this period, and the following diet was taken at the end of the 14 days:

Breakfast—2 coddled eggs.
　　　　　　2 pieces hard, dry, brown toast.
　　　　　　1 dish cooked apple sauce without sugar.

Lunch—　　2 raw apples with 1 ounce of either pecan or almond nuts, together with a glass of water.

Dinner—　 1 small piece of broiled steak.
　　　　　　1 dish of spinach.
　　　　　　Raw celery.
　　　　　　1 dish cooked prunes (without sugar).

"This diet was taken for two days, after which the dinner was changed to the following:

Dinner— Choice of one of the following: lean beef, mutton, chicken, turkey, rabbit or fish.

Choice of two of the following cooked vegetables: celery, asparagus, spinach, Swiss chard, summer squash, small green string beans, kale, lettuce, chayotes, oyster plant, beet tops, French artichoke, mustard greens, turnip tops.

Raw celery as much as desired.

Choice of the following cooked fruits: prunes, pears, apricots, figs, raisins, apple sauce or baked apple.

"Vigorous exercises were recommended morning and night, and long walks advised. The patient has remained in perfect health since that time, and has had no return of epilepsy. I am citing this case in support of my contention that epilepsy is not caused by a meat diet, but is always produced by a toxemia originating in the large colon from the fermentation of different foods, and more especially from starches and sugars. Other diseases, of course, may be produced by excessive meat eating, especially if meat is used in wrong combination with other foods, yet I do not believe it is a factor to be considered in the cause of epilepsy. After health is restored to normal, nuts and cheese may be substituted for meat by those who have a religious or ethical objection to the use of fleshy foods."

RAPID HEALING FOODS
FOR THE NERVES

Apple cider vinegar can reportedly stop any headache—even migraines—within a half hour. Dose: a little apple cider vinegar in water daily. Or, place equal parts of apple cider vinegar and water in a steamer, cover your head and inhale it. Honey can cure migraines. One woman takes a tablespoon of honey as soon as she feels a migraine coming on. If the headache returns, she takes a second dose and three glasses of water. Her headache disappears completely and doesn't return. Raw vegetables can relieve migraine headaches. One man suffered severe migraines for 10 years. Then he discovered that when he began to eat lots of raw vegetables with every meal—tomatoes, cabbage, cucumbers, radishes and more—his migraine headaches stopped.

Soybean lecithin can relieve migraines. One woman says that if she takes an extra-large dose of lecithin as soon as the headache starts, it disappears right then and there. Just taking some daily makes headaches much milder. One woman who uses the same method says she has not taken one Fiorenal tablet since starting. Spinach is loaded with enzymes that break down headache-causing chemicals. Eat all the spinach you can, say medical experts, and avoid spicy or fermented foods, alcohol, chocolate and dairy products.

Elderberry juice can relieve spasms of the face, with pain of a stabbing or throbbing nature, known as tic douloureux or trigeminal neuralgia. In 1914, a Prague doctor cured 48 cases with pure elderberry juice, 20 grams. Some were cured with only one dose. Others after a few days. Adding 20 percent port wine speeds the healing. Elderberry juice can also cure sciatica. A Norwegian doctor combined 10 grams of port wine with 30 grams of elderberry juice, and discovered that acute cases of sciatica were cured in as little as one day.

Goldenseal can bring immediate relief from shingles. This common herb is available at most health stores in powder or capsule form. One woman dissolved some in water, and applied it to the area several times a day and before bed. This worked after a doctor's lotion failed. "Almost immediately," she says, "the shingles started drying up." In two weeks, they were completely gone. She also drank 1 capsule with warm water an hour before each meal (reportedly a safer dose is ⅓ teaspoon daily, no more).

Buckwheat cake has been used to halt MS (multiple sclerosis). In one reported case, a young M.D. was able to halt the progress of his own MS by eating buckwheat cakes. He quickly saw his symptoms (muscle jerking, tremors, lack of coordination) disappear, and never return. Vinegar can relieve MS symptoms. One woman with multiple sclerosis said her whole left side was weak and her left leg was so stiff at times she could not go up and down the stairs. Nothing seemed to help until she read that a doctor said vinegar builds strong muscles. She started drinking about an ounce a day mixed with honey. In a week, her feet stopped trembling, but she still felt weak. So she started drinking a half glass a day. The improvement was dramatic. She has most of her strength back now, she says.

Safflower oil and sunflower seeds can relieve MS. Researchers say sunflower seed oil (2 tablespoons, twice a day) seems to prolong quiescent periods. One man with MS was blind in one eye, numb in various parts of his body, with poor coordination and impaired speech. He was hospitalized and unable to work for a year. He read that safflower oil, sunflower seeds and vitamin E might help. Since using them, his sight returned and all symptoms disappeared with no relapse. His doctor says to keep it up. He no longer needs medication for leg cramps.

Wheat germ oil has relieved muscular dystrophy. We are told that 25 children afflicted with this crippling and wasting disease were given wheat germ oil daily, plus vitamins C and B. Every child improved, and there was one complete recovery. Wheat germ oil has relieved cerebral palsy. A young child suffered from cerebral palsy, which caused spastic paralysis of his arms and legs (wild, jerky movements) and affected his speech. Someone suggested wheat germ oil, which has been found to bring relief, along with vitamin, mineral and protein supplements. In a month, his withered muscles firmed up, and he could soon run and play like any normal child.

Sunflower seed oil has cured paralysis stemming from polyneuritis. In this ailment, a virus causes white blood cells to stop attacking germs and attack healthy nerve tissue instead. A young girl was almost totally paralyzed, and could not move her arms or legs. Doctors said it was permanent. When her parents heard this virus was halted by sunflower oil, they bought a bottle from a health food store and gave her a teaspoonful, three times a day. In 48 hours she began to move. Her father doubled the dose. Soon she could run and play, like any normal child, and today seems completely cured.

QUICK RUNDOWN OF FOODS
THAT HAVE BEEN USED
IN TREATING SPECIFIC AILMENTS

Cerebral Palsy

wheat germ
  oil
multiple vi-
  tamin sup-
  plements

Epilepsy

almonds
apples
apricots
asparagus
beef
beet tops
chayotes
celery
chicken
eggs
figs
fish
grapefruit
kale
lettuce
olive oil
oyster plant
pears

pecans
prunes
rabbit
raisins
steak
string beans
summer squash
Swiss chard
toast
turkey
water

Facial Spasms

elderberry juice
port wine

Migraine

apple cider
  vinegar
cabbage
cucumbers
honey
radishes
soybean lecithin
spinach
tomatoes

Multiple Sclerosis

buckwheat cake
safflower oil
sunflower seeds
vinegar
vitamin E

Muscular Dystrophy

wheat germ oil
vitamin C
vitamin B

Sciatica

elderberry juice
port wine

Shaking Palsy

fresh fruits
nuts
raw vegetables
unprocessed, mild
  cheese

Shingles

goldenseal

12

Rapid Healing Foods for Female Organs!

Practically every ache and pain a woman experiences can be traced to wrong eating habits, resulting in an accumulation of toxic waste material in the body, and a good cleansing diet can relieve symptoms that range from headache, constipation and fatigue, to cramps, nausea, itching, discharge, painful breasts, non-malignant lumps, bumps, menstrual and menopausal problems and much more, say drugless doctors.

Nausea in pregnancy, for example, can be completely and permanently relieved in three to 10 days—with a cleansing diet—so that there will be no more discomfort for the remainder of the pregnancy. And that is simply because nausea is a signal the body wants to clean house.

Think about it. There is rebellion in the stomach; it rejects food, by vomiting if necessary. Nature is trying to provide a clean house for the baby. Many women think they need plenty of "good food" during pregnancy, but the body throws it back. Nausea—revulsion at even the sight, odor or thought of food—is nature's way of telling you to stop eating for awhile. "Go to bed

169

and keep warm," says one drugless doctor. "My experience has shown that three to 10 days are enough to enable the body to put its house in order and there is no more nausea and vomiting throughout the remainder of the pregnancy ... In ordinary cases of morning sickness three to four days of fasting (cleansing) are sufficient to restore comfort and enable the woman to eat without distress ... I have never had a patient fail to become comfortable in a few days (without any suppressing drugs)."

When a pregnant woman first begins to feel nausea, he says, she should voluntarily cease eating at once. Neither she nor the child will be hurt by ceasing to eat, for a short while. A few days of abstinence in the early days of pregnancy (nothing but water or fruit juices) will help relieve morning sickness. A period of light feeding of fruits and uncooked vegetables should follow the fast for a few days before the normal diet is resumed. Pregnant women eat too much, says this doctor. They overeat on proteins. They need good protein, but not in large quantities, he says. Their greatest need is for fruits and green, nonstarchy vegetables.

OTHER SYMPTOMS RELIEVED

Fasting has enabled many women to conceive after years of sterility, says this doctor. Many of these women gave a history of menstrual irregularities, profuse flow, severe cramps, clots, soreness of the breasts and similar symptoms that indicate endocrine gland imbalance, inflammation of the ovaries or womb and nervous difficulties. Others gave a history of metritis (inflammation of the uterus) with a more or less chronic vaginal discharge, which is highly acid and destroys sperm. These are the types of cases that are most easily helped to good health by a cleansing diet or fast. It will also prevent miscarriages, he says. A woman who had 28 miscarriages, after a fast of 10 days and a greatly improved diet, became pregnant and had a normal, healthy baby. Another who was childless after 10 years of marriage and suffered agonies with each menstruation, taking to bed and relieving her pain with drugs, was permanently relieved of pain on menstruation after a 10-day fast, and she too became pregnant shortly afterward and had a healthy baby.

LUMPS, BUMPS AND GROWTHS DISAPPEAR IN MANY CASES!

Cancer is a word that strikes terror in the heart of every woman, and no woman should take any chances. By all means, have regular, thorough checkups, and follow your doctor's advice. But be sure you have all the most accurate tests available, including biopsy. Drugless doctors have seen many non-malignant lumps, bumps and growths disappear in as little as three days to two weeks, others from three to six weeks, on a cleansing diet or fast.

Just as fasting causes the body to use up excess fat, in dieting, so it causes the breakdown, by the process of autolysis, of non-malignant growths or tumors. In like manner, dropsical swellings, edematous swellings, deposits and infiltrations are absorbed, nonusable portions excreted.

One woman had a fibroid tumor of the uterus about the size of a lemon. A doctor recommended immediate surgery to remove her uterus and ovaries. This woman refused the operation and resorted to a cleansing diet. With this method, the tumor was soon dissolved, and disappeared, and her organs were saved. Another woman had a uterine fibroid about the size of a grapefruit. The tumor was completely dissolved in 28 days on a cleansing diet. Thousands of women have been saved from operations by cleansing diets, which work on the same principle as the removal of fat on a reducing diet, says one doctor.

UTERINE FIBROIDS DISAPPEAR

Another drugless doctor claimed: "I do not believe that surgical measures are necessary or advisable in the treatment of fibroid tumors. There are several factors which must be considered (in) cure without surgery. The immediate cause of every one of these growths is the congestion in the uterus of morbid material deposited from a sluggish circulation ... However, I find that a long (cleansing diet) will absorb this enlargement and toughened growth, so that (with warm baths and a few other simple corrective measures) the uterus can be made to remain fairly normal.

"A young woman, 28, had a large fibroid tumor partially protruding from the vagina, and about the size of a large grapefruit. The stomach and intestines were prolapsed (sagging) and lying upon the fibroid, which was being pushed downward by the weight. An orange juice fast was started, using a glass of orange juice three times daily, together with a glass of water. Although the patient weighed only 112 pounds at the start of treatment, this fast was continued for 28 days, reducing the weight to 92 pounds. By this time about three-fourths of the tumor had been removed by the absorbing power of the fast treatment. The patient was put on a milk diet at this point, taking a glass of raw milk every hour until 3 quarts were taken each day. This was gradually increased to 6 quarts daily, and the patient's weight was brought up from 92 pounds at the end of the fast to 128 pounds at the end of 60 days.

"She then started a general diet, using calisthenic exercises and taking long walks, and appeared to be in good health, although the fibroid growth had not entirely disappeared ... After six months in all of treatment she was married, and during the first month of married life all signs of the tumor entirely disappeared. She is now in perfect health, with the tissues of her uterus in as healthy a condition as it would be possible to find in one who had never suffered from a female disorder.

"A woman, 54, had been examined by the leading surgeons of (San Francisco), who advised an operation for the removal of a large fibroid tumor which almost completely filled the lower abdomen. She waited several months after being first told of her serious condition, until every one of the surgeons who had advised an operation refused to operate upon her, claiming that she could not live through it because of a heart condition which had developed through the tremendous pressure of the tumor. A close friend happened to call upon her, who had been a patient of mine, and had been cured of a fibroid tumor. She telegraphed to me asking my advice, stating that the patient's pulse beat was then 160 per minute, and that the doctors gave her no hope of recovery. I telegraphed as follows:

> "Put patient on water fast at once, allowing her to drink water only when very thirsty. She may add a few drops of lemon to the water. Two enemas daily. Two epsom salt sponge baths daily."

"These instructions were followed strictly, being easily interpreted by the friend who had been my patient, and who had been under a similar treatment. After two weeks of this fast the pulse had reduced to a little under 100, and the patient was strong enough and had improved enough in every way to be able to take the train trip of 500 miles to Los Angeles. Her fast was continued for two weeks (with various local treatments) but because of lack of funds she returned to San Francisco. When she left the pulse was 90, and the tumor had been reduced, according to her estimate, to about one-third of the original size. She was then placed upon the following diet:

Breakfast—Whites of 2 eggs.
　　　　　3 pieces of brown, thin toast.
　　　　　5 Senna prunes.
Lunch—　One of the following fruits: pears, peaches, grapes, apples, apricots, plums, or a glass of orange juice.
Dinner—　Lean beef or mutton.
　　　　　1 nonstarchy vegetable.
　　　　　Raw celery or tomatoes.

"This diet was continued strictly for three months, and she reported to me by letter, claiming there was a gradual improvement in her health in every way, with a slow decrease in the size of the tumor. She was then put upon a diet which gave her a larger quantity of food value, and continued on this diet for over two years, with occasional fasting periods which she took of her own accord. She was advised to take treatments at her home with hot applications over the abdomen, and three times a week was advised to take a hot bath containing a large quantity of epsom salt. She was also instructed to take two hot douches each day, and vigorous calisthenic exercises twice daily. At the end of two and a half years from the time I first gave her the advice by telegraph, she again presented herself to the same surgeons who had refused to operate on her, and they pronounced her perfectly well, and said there was no sign of any fibroid growth."

PAINFUL MENSTRUATION

The menstrual life of a woman is as varied as climate and racial development. Among all the primitive races the act of menstruation is performed without discomfort, and has as its object the ejection of an unfertile egg of microscopic size, which requires very little fluid or effort. Civilized woman, however, eating large quantities of starchy, mucus-forming foods, has developed the habit of having a copious discharge of blood once every 28 days to accomplish the same object. If pain is present, it is due to some congestion in the womb or ovaries. An osteopathic drugless doctor describes his treatment, in this case:

"An unmarried woman, 27 suffered from backache in the lower part of the back, and had great pain at the start of each menstrual period, so that she was confined to her bed two or three days at a time. Her back hurt off and on at other times of the month, too. Examination showed a prolapsed uterus (sagging out of place) and lying upon the rectum. She was given a fast (a cleansing diet), at first taking three meals a day of cherries (taking all she desired each time) and using at least one glass of water with each cherry meal. This was continued for two weeks. On the tenth day, her menstruation started with less pain than at any other time in her life. After two weeks, the fast was changed to plain water for an additional five days. In both these fasts two enemas daily were taken to ensure a complete cleansing of the lower bowel. Following the water fast, she was put on the following diet:

> Breakfast—
> 1 dish of whole wheat mush made from whole wheat, coarse ground, cooked slowly for one hour, and seasoned with butter or cream.
>
> Lunch—   Choice of one of the following fruits: apples, figs, cherries or peaches, together with 2 ounces of pecan or almond nuts.
>
> Dinner— Choice of one of the following proteins: lean beef or mutton, fish, chicken, turkey, rabbit.
>
> Choice of two cooked nonstarchy vegetables and choice of salad vegetables.
>
> Dessert: Stewed fruit.

"Treatment was continued for several months with steady improvement (with exercises for developing the abdominal muscles) ... Shortly after this the patient was married, and after three months of married life a re-examination showed the uterus in normal position, with no fibroid growth evident. About a month after marriage the backache entirely disappeared, and two menstruations have been passed without a sign of any symptoms of pain or disorder ... The change in her condition after marriage was so rapid, that I am forced to believe that in this case, as in many others, the adoption of normal sexual habits had a great deal to do with the cure."

SCANTY OR IRREGULAR MENSTRUATION

This condition may be caused by anemia or some form of gastro-intestinal disturbance which produces pressure upon the womb or ovaries, either by impacted feces or excess gas pressure. The anemia must be cured by proper dietary changes, and the correction of all habits which produce the faulty metabolism. If low blood pressure exists, it may take several months before a normal menstrual flow is established, occurring at the proper intervals. In other toxic states such as diabetes, these ailments must be relieved first. In cases of valvular leakage of the heart, the menses may cease until the heart is functioning properly. A doctor reported the following cases.

"A married woman, 37, had suffered headaches since childhood. Her menstrual periods varied from six weeks to eight, 11 and 20 weeks. On one occasion, six months passed, and at another time 20 months passed without any sign of the menses. During this last period a valvular heart trouble developed and she could not climb one flight of stairs or use her arms in housework. She had been told by three different doctors that at her age nothing could be done to correct this condition. She had been examined by many physicians in different parts of the country, and had been treated by them with medicines, electricity, osteopathy, etc. When the patient came to me for treatment she had not menstruated for 10 weeks, and was suffering from chronic gastritis which she had had for several years.

"She was advised to take an orange juice fast (a cleansing diet), and continued this for 30 days, using the juice of about six oranges daily, with a plentiful supply of water. After about two weeks of this fast, menstruation started, and has continued to occur at regular periods every four weeks for the last seven years. The chronic condition of gastritis was, of course, cured by the fast, which was followed by judicious dieting. The headaches stopped after the second day of the fast, and have never occurred since. The patient is now 44 years of age, and has every appearance of being in perfect health."

PROFUSE MENSTRUATION

This disorder usually occurs with women who are passing through the change of life or menopause. It may be caused by lack of fibrogen, a clotting factor, in the blood, or by lacerations or tears in the womb left from childbirth (which can often only be stopped by surgical repair), or from irritation produced by polyps or small growths inside the uterus (which are removed in a simple operation called curettement). A doctor reported the following case, cured without drugs or surgery.

"A woman, 45, was menstruating steadily for three months. Several doctors told her an operation was absolutely necessary to remove tumors in the womb, which they said existed. Upon examination I could not discover the presence of any such tumors, and immediately put the patient on a water fast (a cleansing diet), which was taken for four days, after which the patient took the following diet:

Six times daily she dissolved the contents of one package of jello or gelatin in a pint of hot water, and immediately drank it.

"This was taken for three days, but on the first day of the gelatin diet menstruation ceased entirely. However, the gelatin was continued for two days more, after which the patient took a well-balanced diet, using a dish of jello every other day for several weeks. Four weeks after menstruation ceased, the menses again started, and continued normally for about four days. They have since appeared at the regular 28-day intervals for over two years. It has never been necessary to take any further treatment, as the patient seems to be perfectly normal in every way."

"MENSTRUAL" HEADACHES VANISH

A woman, 34, had suffered from headaches in the back of her head ever since puberty. They occurred a day or two before the start of menstruation, disappearing for a day during the period, and recurring just at the end of it. They also occurred at different times during the month. She went to a drugless doctor, who noticed her sagging stomach and intestines, and a prolapsed uterus. A few days before her period, she was told to start a fast or cleansing diet, using only plain water. Two enemas a day were taken. The menses started without a sign of headache. "Relief from this kind of headache caused by uterine congestion is usually brought about as quickly as the bowels are completely emptied by enemas, as this frees the circulation to and coming from the uterus," said the doctor reporting this case.

The fast was continued for 10 days, and the patient was then put on a general diet. Suitable exercises were recommended for strengthening the abdomen and the uterus gradually moved back to a normal position. The normal sexual impulse returned, and a few months later this patient became pregnant for the first time in her married life of 16 years, and gave birth to a strong boy. She never had a recurrence of any form of headache.

PROLAPSUS, OR SAGGING OF ORGANS

Most of the vital organs of the body are attached by the ligaments to the spine, and if man walked on all fours the organs would hang from the spine in the same way as they do in any of the monkey family. Primitive man no doubt assumed a posture similar to that of the apes most of the time, but developed an upright position as it became more convenient to carry things in his hands. As a result, those organs attached to the spine have, by degrees, sagged lower down in the abdomen. Where great weakness exists, or the muscles of the body are allowed to degenerate by disuse, this prolapsus has become more and more pronounced, so that one organ is lying on top of the other, and all are pressed further down into the basin of the pelvis. Those who are forced to work where they are constantly standing will almost always have an abnormal prolapsus of stomach and intestines.

In women, the uterus is usually out of normal position. One doctor says, "From time to time I have had patients who were classical dancers, and in every case I have examined so far the stomach and intestines have been prolapsed several inches." This doctor reports the following cases.

"A woman, 68, had a uterus so prolapsed as to protrude several inches outside of the vagina, with the result that an oil bandage had to be worn to hold it up sufficiently to enable the patient to walk. An operation had been advised by many physicians, but the patient would not consent. The physician who advised the operation said that apparently there had been a tearing loose of some of the ligaments attached to the womb when the last child was born, which happened when the woman was 42 years of age, and that because of this tearing she could never expect to have the womb return to its normal place by any means other than surgery, where the organ would be sewed to the abdominal wall...

"The patient was put on a fast (a cleansing diet) of orange juice and water, taking the juice of an orange every two hours with a glass of water, and taking two enemas daily. This was continued for 32 days, during which time the patient lost nearly 30 pounds of weight. After the fast the following diet was prescribed:

Breakfast—Glass of orange juice and a glass of water.
Lunch—   2 coddled eggs.
          Choice of 1 nonstarchy cooked vegetable.
          Choice of 1 salad vegetable.
          1 stewed fruit.
Dinner—   1 protein food, selected from the following: lean
          beef or mutton, fish, turkey, chicken or rabbit.
          2 nonstarchy vegetables.
          1 or more salad vegetables.

"After a few days of this diet the patient was instructed to take calisthenic exercises (see pages 180-182), especially those to be practiced while lying on the back. Her diet was gradually increased, and she was instructed to take short walks several times during the day.

"After six months, I again examined the patient, with x-rays, and found that the stomach and intestines had nearly resumed their normal position, but the uterus still protruded slightly from the vagina. The patient seemed discouraged. I advised her that no matter how slow the cure seemed, she should continue to do exactly as she had been doing, and that eventually the organ would be raised enough to make her comfortable. She was finally persuaded to continue the exercise and diet treatment at home.

"At the end of a month, when she returned to me for examination, I found that the uterus had returned to a perfectly normal position, and that her stomach and intestines had also been raised to their proper places. The preparatory treatments during the first six months, it should be explained, were strengthening and preparing the muscles of the abdomen for what might be called their new duties, so that quite suddenly during the seventh month the uterus returned to its normal position. She has remained perfectly well for over six years, and is now 74 years of age. From my experience I am satisfied that a woman of advanced years can develop her abdominal muscles just as easily as a young girl. These muscles are actually still undeveloped, in such cases, have never before been used—and hence are not worn out. Let me cite another case.

"A woman, 32, one of the best known classical dancers on the American stage, had suffered from prolapsus of the uterus, secretly, for many years, and had been forced at times to wear a certain kind of metal pessary, which is a device used for holding up the uterus in the worst stages of prolapsus. Sometimes the trouble became so pronounced that she was unable to continue her theatrical engagements. As dancing is so frequently recommended as a good exercise it had always puzzled her as to how this prolapsus could exist with the vigorous training she had undergone, and the constant practice of dancing exercises.

"I assured her that those muscles of the abdomen which were used by the body to hold the vital organs in position were not sufficiently exercised by a classical dancer to be able to overcome the violent jars the body was constantly subjected to during certain parts of the dances, where leaps, etc., were indulged in. I showed her how her back muscles and the muscles of the thigh and the calf were very well developed, but that the abdominal muscles were so weak that while she was standing in an attitude of repose there was such a prolapsus of the abdominal viscera that her abdomen protruded several inches beyond the normal.

"After going through a treatment with a short fast and diet regime, she was instructed to take abdominal exercises, and she continued taking them three times daily for about three months, which happened to be her vacation period. By the end of that time the uterus was in its normal position, and the abdominal muscles were so strong that there was no protrusion or sagging of the abdomen, while another x-ray examination at that time disclosed the fact that her stomach and intestines had returned to their normal position. She felt fine in every way, and was relieved of many symptoms such as headaches and nausea and pains in the legs from which she had previously suffered because of her disorder ... she has remained perfectly well and without any sign of prolapsus for more than five years."

EXERCISES FOR STRENGTHENING ABDOMINAL MUSCLES

These simple body movements—done mostly while lying on the back, on the floor—if persisted in twice daily, will so develop the abdominal muscles and those of the entire front of the body, that no matter how much out of position the organs may have sagged they will gradually be brought back into their normal places, says this doctor. In this way the stomach, intestines and uterus are held up in such a position that they can function properly, and one will not interfere with the free action of another.

Lying on Back

1. Extend hands over head. Raise upper body—keeping knees stiff. Touch your legs as far toward the feet as possible with your fingertips.

2. Raise knees alternately to chest and return. Raise knees together to chest and return.

3. Raise and lower legs alternately—keeping the knees stiff and toes pointed downward.

4. Raise and lower both legs together—keeping knees stiff and toes pointed downward.

5. Raise right leg to right angle with body, keeping the toes pointed downward—then change position of right and left legs vigorously, without allowing the heels to touch the floor. Try to breathe naturally during this exercise.

6. Extend arms on floor at right angles to body—palms pointing downward—keep the arms and shoulders in this position and bring the right foot over and touch the left hand—twisting the body and bending the knee as much as necessary to do so. Return to original position and repeat with left foot, touching the right hand.

7. Arms overhead—raise both arms and legs together, at the same time keeping knees stiff and touching the legs as far down toward the feet as possible.

8. Hands clasped behind head—slowly raise the arms, head and shoulders as high as possible, attempting to come to a sitting position.

These simple movements will gradually raise any prolapsed (sagging) organs to the normal position. If you start taking these exercises, go through the entire list first of all, doing the easy ones a greater number of times than the more difficult ones, and as strength and ability develop, gradually eliminate the easier exercises altogether and do only those which you found hard in the first place, says this doctor. You will find that as your muscular power increases you can concentrate your time on only a few of the exercises taken from each position, and if you will do these as vigorously as you can, after two or three weeks you will find that 10 minutes' time daily will be sufficient for you.

Lying Face Downward

The exercises taken while lying face downward develop the different muscles attached to the spine, and such development will hold the vertebrae of the spine in their proper place.

With simple body movements of this kind, says one drugless doctor, the spinal muscles may be so strongly developed in a few months' time that neither the osteopath nor the chiropractor will be able to find a subluxated (partially dislocated) vertebra.

These subluxated vertebrae, which pinch upon the nerves issuing from the spine, are the direct or indirect cause of different diseases brought about by the shutting off of the nerve supply to the various parts of the body served by these particular nerves, say drugless doctors.

1. Lying face downward, clasp hands behind neck—then raise head, shoulders and elbows as high as possible, at the same time raising both legs, keeping knees stiff.

2. Raise and lower right and left legs alternately—keeping the knees stiff and bending the legs backward at the hips.

3. Arms extended straight over the head—raise the arms, head and shoulders, at the same time raising the legs and keeping the knees stiff.

4. Hands pointing out straight overhead—raise arms, shoulders and head, also raise the legs, keeping the knees stiff. Inhale as you raise to this position, and exhale upon returning to original position.

Next, separate the hands to the distance of about 2 feet, and raise and lower as before.

Then extend the hands straight out from the shoulders and repeat as before. (Subsequently, reverse this exercise, going back to the original position.)

In item 4, if you wish, as strength of back muscles develops, you may try this advanced exercise: change the position of the arms only a few inches at a time. For example, in this exercise you have only four different positions of the arms, but this can easily be increased to 15 or 20 by making a slight change in the position of the arms.

5. Arms extended straight out from side, with palms pointing downward—bring the right foot over and touch the left hand, bending the knee and twisting the body as much as possible, but keeping the chest and arms flat on the floor. Return to original position, and repeat with the left foot, touching the right hand.

Take these exercises both in the morning and evening, slowly at first, doing each one two or three times, and increasing as you are able. While these exercises are being practiced for the development of the back muscles, it is advisable at the same time to keep up osteopathic or chiropractic treatments until the muscles attached to the spine have developed sufficient strength through the exercising to hold the vertebrae in the normal position.

RAPID HEALING FOODS FOR WOMEN'S AILMENTS

Garlic can relieve vaginal infections. One woman says: "For five years I suffered from an agonizing vaginal yeast infection. I saw a total of four doctors ... They gave me every remedy from purple dye to strong antibiotics ... After reading that garlic acts like an antibiotic, I began to take fresh garlic cut up, and later on, manufactured garlic pills. I have found that, like an antibiotic, when I discontinue the garlic, the infection starts again. But there are two distinct advantages of taking the garlic (combined with vinegar douches) over the doctor-prescribed antibiotics. It is much cheaper and there are no side effects."

Acidophilus yogurt may relieve a monilia (candida) infection. One woman suffered with this for seven years and numerous gynecologists could not cure it. Then she tried frequent doses of acidophilus culture in pill form (available at health foods stores), plus eating yogurt instead of sour cream. This cured her monilia.

Fresh acidophilus yogurt can relieve vaginitis-cystitis. One woman suffered with this for 13 years. Nothing doctors gave her helped and the condition worsened. The infection from the vagina would travel to the bladder, causing discomfort and frequent urination. When she heard that relief was possible by inserting freshy made acidophilus yogurt directly into the vagina by means of a plastic applicator available at drugstores, she tried it. "Almost immediately my bladder symptoms abated and much of the vaginal irritation I had experienced for so long disappeared." After three months, she said, "I have been delighted to find that I can travel, work and engage in activities without the constant desire to urinate."

Garlic is said to relieve menstrual and menopausal problems, including hot flashes, depression, irritability, anxiety, nausea, headache, tiredness, bloating, swelling of the extremities, dizziness, morning sickness, premenstrual tension, itching, leukorrhea, arthritis and more. A proven emmenagogue, it stimulates the menstrual flow. It can relieve menstrual cramps, as well. One woman says: "I've always had menstrual cramps constantly, the first two days. But ever since taking garlic (about three months) I have hardly any. It's hard to believe, but it is the only thing I'm taking that I didn't take before that time. Now on each day of menstruation I take four or five garlic pills, available at any health food store. I take two or three every day and, as said before, four or five on those difficult days."

Red raspberry tea can relieve labor pains and miscarriage. One doctor reports, in a good many cases labor has been easy and painless. One woman had four miscarriages and several doctors said she could never be a mother. A friend suggested this tea which she drank every morning during pregnancy. She gave birth to a normal baby, and in 18 months had another. In many cases, labor has been practically painless. So painless, in fact, that another woman who drank red raspberry tea was reading a paper only a few minutes before her baby was born.

Foods that seem to relieve anemia include eggs, meat, vegetables, beef liver, kidney beans, apricots, whole wheat bread, parsely, spinach, beet greens and garlic. Kelp relieves anemia. When 400 obstetrical patients were given kelp tablets, within six to eight weeks on three a day, the hemoglobin levels of their blood rose 85 percent. In all patients studied, there was a spectacular drop in the incidence of colds. Those with a history of miscarriage had normal pregnancies. Other foods that relieve anemia include honey, peaches, prunes, raisins, parsnips, cauliflower, beets, blackberries, pineapples, sweet potatoes and grapes.

Garlic, kelp and seafoods may relieve a sluggish thyroid with symptoms of sluggishness, overweight, headaches, fatigue, weakness, and chilly or clammy hands and feet. Also, in cases of stubborn overweight, fennel tea can help you shed unwanted pounds. One lady reported that she slimmed down 70 pounds by drinking four cups each day. She did not follow a strict diet but just cut down a little on starches and sweets. Besides losing weight, an old eye discomfort (bright light hurt her eyes) disappeared. Others who could not lose weight, even on strict diets, found that the addition of fennel caused weight to drop steadily. Once normal they could be fairly liberal in their eating habits without gaining (it helps digestion, too). Tea made of cleavers also seems to cause weight loss. One woman used it to lose 32 pounds in six months and has not put back an ounce. In this case it may take about a month to show effects.

QUICK RUNDOWN OF FOODS
THAT HAVE BEEN USED
IN TREATING SPECIFIC AILMENTS

Anemia	kelp kidney beans	*Labor Pain or* *Miscarriages*
apricots	liver	
beef	meat	red raspberry tea
beet greens	parsley	
beets	parsnips	*Menstrual and*
blackberries	peaches	*Menopausal*
cauliflower	pineapples	*Symptoms*
eggs	prunes	blueberries
garlic	raisins	garlic
grapes	spinach	parsley
honey	sweet potatoes	raspberries

Menstrual Cramps

blackberries
garlic
parsley
raspberries

Menstrual Headaches

blueberries
parsley
water (plain
water fast and
two enemas
daily a few
days before
period, see
page 177).

Nausea in Pregnancy

fruit juice or
water fast (see
page 170)
light meals of
fresh fruit,
uncooked non-
starchy
vegetables, see
page 170.

Painful Menstruation

cherry fast (three
meals a day, as
much as
desired, with a
glass of water
each time) for
two weeks,
followed by
general diet,
see page 174-5:

apples
almonds
chicken
exercises (see
page 180-2)
figs
fish
lean beef
mutton
nonstarchy
vegetables
peaches
pecans
rabbit
salad vegetables
stewed fruit
turkey
whole wheat
mush

Profuse Menstruation

blackberries
fast on jello or
gelatin in a
pint of water,
six times daily
for three days,
followed by
balanced diet,
see page 176.

Prolapsed Uterus

orange juice and
water
fast .
followed by
general diet
and abdominal
exercise (see
page 180-2):
chicken
coddled eggs

fish
lean beef
mutton
nonstarchy
vegetables
rabbit
salad vegetables
stewed fruit
turkey

Scanty or Irregular Menstruation

orange juice fast
(six oranges
daily) and
plenty of water,
see page 175-6.
carrots

Sluggish Thyroid

garlic
kelp
seafoods

Stubborn Overweight

fennel tea
cleavers

Vaginal Infections

acidophilus
yogurt
(freshly made,
as suppository)
garlic
vinegar douches

13

Rapid Healing Foods for Male Organs!

The most common problem among men is "prostate trouble." The mysterious prostate is a ball-shaped organ, entirely different in function and location from the testicles. It surrounds the urethra (tube leading from bladder to penis) like a "muff" around a gas or water pipe. It seems protective, so that this tube cannot be torn by swelling of the bladder or penis. It looks something like a nut with a tube running through it. This gland secretes fluid into which sperm—from the testicles—is ejaculated during sex. You never know it exists unless it swells, choking off the tube. This is caused by:

1. A vitamin or mineral deficiency (especially zinc).
2. Lack of alkaline salts present especially in green vegetables.
3. Too much sex, which irritates the gland.
4. Too little sex, which causes fluid to collect, coagulate and irritate.
5. Too little exercise, which causes fluid to collect in the prostate, causing enlargement, even prostate stones.

6. Stones traveling down from kidneys or bladder.
7. Overweight, which causes congestion and pressure in the pelvic organs.
8. Wrong food combinations that constipate.
9. Germs, including venereal germs, which travel up the penis.

Irritation from retained urine is painful. The urine is highly acid, and it burns. The swollen prostate, choking off the urine, causes a feeling of fullness, difficulty starting a stream, the need to squeeze in order to start, a feeling you have more left that won't come out, dribbling long afterward (especially when straining, coughing, or excited), frequent night rising to urinate, without result, increased sexual desire. All these are symptoms which sufferers have reported.

There are other contributing causes of prostate irritation. One is the habit of lingering in bed, with a full bladder, in the morning. This causes a somewhat painful erection that is very uncomfortable. The bladder—filled with urine, presses against the base of the penis, causing a very hard erection that won't go down until the urine is voided, which is somewhat awkward and painful in that position. Experienced by every man on those mornings when you're too lazy to get up, it can be extremely embarrassing, and avoided only if you happen to wake up before the bladder is full. The congestion and pressure on internal organs is obvious. An additional irritation is attempting sexual activity in this condition, or simply delaying urination for long periods of time.

Another cause of prostate irritation is the deliberate withholding or delaying of orgasm during sex, to prolong pleasure, or prolong your erection. This is a very common cause of prostate irritation that starts in boys at age 12 or 13. If a habit develops in delaying orgasm for unreasonably long periods, two hours, four hours, an entire day or evening, trying to control your breaking point, letting it subside, perhaps even going to sleep without ever having ejaculated, it can cause serious trouble. In the beginning, this fluid re-absorbs. But after a while, it collects. It is not good "practice" for pleasing yourself or anyone else. Your prostate can *enlarge*. Your capacity is increased, but you can die of uremic poisoning.

THE FINAL EFFECT

Of all the agony caused by an enlarged prostate, the worst is complete stoppage of urine. Repeated irritation causes the gland to swell, choking off the urinary tube that it literally surrounds, like a doughnut. This usually happens at some advanced point (usually middle or late life), but it can and does occur at any age from 25 on up. Urine backs up in the bladder. The bladder swells to enormous size. The kidneys are overloaded. Uremic poisoning occurs, with fever, chills and death—if the bladder is not drained immediately. To do this, a doctor inserts a tube (catheter) through the penis into the bladder, and lets it drain. He leaves the tube inserted, for further drainage into a bag which is strapped to your leg. You may go home this way, and have to endure it for quite some time.

With repeated attacks, surgery is often recommended as a last resort. The gland is not removed in most cases. Instead, the inner lining, which has a tendency to swell, is "carved" out, rendering the man sterile (unable to cause pregnancy). He can still have erections and orgasms, but the orgasms are often "dry." Most men say they are not bothered at all by this condition, and their erections and orgasms are just as strong and frequent as before. Some men are bothered, however, and the psychological shock of this often causes impotence (no erection at all). In either case, while immediate relief is felt, post-operative urinary problems eventually return, in the form of infections, irritation, etc., since seminal fluid produced by other glands (without the backup of a prostate for strong ejaculation) is dissipated in the urinary tract, where it may cause congestion.

At present, the better surgeons do not like to remove the prostate. In a man, urine comes through a channel in the prostate—and it is not possible to remove the prostate without cutting the tube leading in and out of it. This tube must be connected directly to the bladder. In this delicate surgery, a perfect connection, avoiding swelling, clotting or blockage—with complete drainage of the bladder—is essential. At one time, prostate removal was very popular. The loss of popularity was due to the high death rate (25 percent). The complication: urinary blockage. For this reason, only in extreme cases, the inner lining is cut out, leaving only a shell through which urine flows. This, too, is a delicate operation, the surgeon entering through the rectum, the penis or pubic area.

For these reasons, most doctors try to avoid surgery. Medical doctors resort to sitz baths, prostate massage and antibiotics at first. Some will tell you to avoid the various causes listed—others say there is no known cause, and have devised operations to remove part of the gland, and various injections or drugs to shrink it. None of these are entirely satisfactory, if causes are ignored.

TOO MUCH SEX

The male body is not built for frequent sexual encounters within a short period of time. With vigorous stimulation, erection can be maintained after orgasm, or experienced again a short time afterward, but it is no accident that "not much is felt" or that the organ feels "anesthetized" or "sore" or that the lower pelvic area feels "heavy" or "very tired." It is telling you to stop. In their quest for pleasure, some men will experience orgasm nearly every day, often several times a day, beyond the point where they are tired, even if it means a dry orgasm. You are courting trouble of a very serious nature by repeated sexual stimulation of this type. Anything beyond reason (withholding more than a half hour, pushing yourself beyond what is natural for you without ache and pain) will lead to trouble, eventually crippling you with urinary problems, infections, excruciating hip, back and leg pains that will not respond to remedies for arthritis or the sciatic nerve, because they are caused by nerves radiating from the prostate area.

NOT ENOUGH SEX

Some sexual release is necessary for every man. The male organs need strong, healthy contraction, with complete empty-ing, on a regular basis—due to a constant build-up in the prostate gland. This fluid seeks release, which may even happen during sleep. Sex or masturbation is a way of controlling this. There is no set rule as to how often this should occur—but it should occur at least once a month. Generally, if left alone, at some time during the month the male organ will elongate and stir, signalling a time for release of accumulated fluid. This may happen more than once a month, but it should not be forced beyond what feels natural.

HOW YOU CAN KEEP YOUR PROSTATE WORKING SMOOTHLY

The cause and cure of prostate trouble lies in avoiding irritating habits. Early or light cases of prostate irritation can be cured completely. In advanced cases, prostate inflammation with swelling or enlargement can often only be controlled. The gland can be reduced in size, temporarily, but once it has enlarged there seems to be a strong tendency for it to enlarge again, on the slightest provocation, such as:

> overeating
> nervous excitement (fear)
> overwork, lack of sleep
> long hours of sitting
> lack of exercise
> excessive use of alcohol or tobacco
> too much or too little sex

A feeling of fullness, difficulty on urination, night-rising and a frequent urge to urinate, burning urine or any symptom of irritation, inflammation or bleeding should be attended to by a doctor at once. The bleeding may be due to simple ulceration caused by highly acid retained urine, or it may be more serious. The doctor can tell if the prostate seems nodular or cancerous. In most cases, symptoms arise from simple prostate irritation, inflammation, enlargement, urethritis (inflammation of the urinary tube) or urinary infection. If infection is present, he will recommend an antibiotic that will clear it up at once, but not permanently if irritating habits are persisted in. In addition, he will usually recommend prostate massages in his office and warm sitz baths when you get home. Anything that causes congestion in the lower abdomen, such as overweight, overeating, constipation, overstimulation, should be avoided.

HOW MASSAGING HELPS

In his book, *A Country Doctor's Common Sense Health Manual*,[1] J. Frank Hurdle, M.D. states: "When your doctor does a rectal examination, he can feel the underneath surface of your prostate gland to see whether it is enlarged or normal in size— the prostate gland normally produces a slight bulge through the front wall of the lower rectum.

"When the prostate gland becomes inflamed, the part of the gland that can be felt through the rectal wall enlarges noticeably and the gland becomes quite tender. Your doctor usually recommends the prostatic massage if this is the case. This is done by 'milking out' the congested prostate. He simply takes his gloved finger and presses down on the gland beginning at the top of the gland and sliding his finger down toward the bottom. This maneuver empties the gland of its excess secretions.

"These secretions are passed into the urethra—the tube leading from the bladder to the outside—where they flow out the penis (you can feel it the instant it's done). The massage also stimulates the circulation in the gland and helps diminish inflammation. If the secretions appear to be infected as well as increased in quantity, your doctor may prescribe rectal irrigations of warm water and perhaps an antibiotic to kill the germs.

"I once talked to a young man in his mid 20's named Hal F., who disproved that 'It's impossible to get too much sex.' He came to my office with his prostate gland engorged to at least twice its normal size. It was so enlarged it was shutting off the flow of urine from his bladder. He had to literally squeeze out his urine and it was acutely painful to do so. In addition, he was running a fever of 101 degrees and had pain in both hips—a common site of pain with prostate trouble ... Hal was having intercourse with as many as five women a week, more than once with some of them. This proved to be his prostate's undoing. It became enlarged, swollen, painful and infected. Hal's case responded to massage, antibiotics and cutting down on his sexual contacts.

---

[1]Parker Publishing Company, Inc., 1975.

Some enlargement of his prostate persisted, so I taught Hal how to do his own prostatic massage.

DO-IT-YOURSELF PROSTATE MASSAGE

"Hal got hold of some rubber finger 'cots' at his drugstore. These are thin rubber tubes that fit snugly over the finger. Three times a week, Hal put one of these finger cots on his right index finger, gently inserted his finger into his rectum about an inch and a half, and milked down his enlarged prostate gland. *Gentleness* during the procedure is essential. If you press down too hard, it is painful and just irritates the prostate further. Done gently once a day or every other day and until the gland comes down to size, however, it can save your prostate from future trouble. Some vaseline on the finger cot may help in passing through the rectum.

"For heat, Hal found that filling an ordinary enema bag with warm water, inserting the nozzle of the enema hose about 2 inches into his rectum and letting the water run in slowly and back out again worked quite well. The object here isn't to 'take an enema,' but just to deliver the warm water to the part of the prostate gland that bulges through the front rectal wall. If the tip isn't inserted too far, the water will run in and then back out into the toilet again."

A CLEANSING DIET CAN
RELIEVE PROSTATE TROUBLE

In some cases, advanced prostatitis can be completely remedied by a fast or cleansing diet. In almost every case—in one or two days—a free flow of urine is restored, and relief is felt, says one drugless doctor. With a fast or cleansing diet, he says:

> "I have seen prostate glands that were as large as baseballs and nearly as hard—cases in which a catheter had to be used (due to complete stoppage of urine)— that were reduced to nearly normal size in a week. The hardness was entirely dissolved, and the victims could urinate freely."

In some cases it does not seem possible to reduce all the enlargement, says this doctor, but it may be reduced so that the urine flows freely, all discomfort in the back, hips and legs (and sometimes lumbago and sciatica, which may be present) are relieved. This is all accomplished by stopping weakening habits, putting the patient to bed and stopping all food for a few days (only water or juices).

This doctor says he has seen patients who were forced to get up as many as 15 to 20 times a night to urinate—able to sleep 13 hours, without getting up, after a few days of fasting. Men who had great difficulty in passing urine were able to do so as freely as when they were boys!

For permanent relief, however, the causes of prostate trouble (as listed previously) must be permanently avoided. After your fast, your diet should include plenty of fresh, green vegetables, fruits, lean beef or lamb, whole grain bread and whole grain cereal. Heavy starches and sweets are to be avoided, as well as all stimulants and highly seasoned foods which irritate the urinary tract. Drink plenty of water to avoid constipation and soothe and cleanse all irritated membranes, says one drugless doctor.

RAPID HEALING FOODS FOR MEN'S PROBLEMS

Sunflower seeds and pumpkin seeds can relieve prostate trouble. One doctor claims he has been curing patients of prostatic trouble by having them eat pumpkin seeds regularly. It seems to stimulate male potency as well, and has an age-delaying effect. Parsley tea is said to relieve prostate trouble. One man says that ever since he started drinking it, he's had relief from both bladder irritation and prostate pressure—relief that has lasted a year. Both these foods are rich in vitamin A, which has a healing and moisturizing effect on the mucous membrane lining of all organs, preventing it from drying up.

Chinese Super Old-Fashioned Compound Herb tea has been used for thousands of years for kidney and bladder problems. It is said to dissolve stones and cause them to be passed. It has brought dramatic relief from prostate trouble. One man who suffered prostate enlargement with infection, pus and low back trouble, drank two bottles of this tea, and the next morning his pains were gone, and he could urinate freely. Others have had the same amazing relief.

Ginseng is said to work miracles in curing impotence. It can be taken as a tea. The roots can be chewed. Long-time sufferers have claimed that after a few weeks, they have felt a sudden surge of power and never had any trouble since.

Fenugreek tea has been recommended for soothing and cleansing the mucous membrane lining of the urinary tract, keeping it free from accumulations of mucus or pus and alleviating any incipient irritations. One expert says he knows of no safer, simpler remedy to avoid prostate irritation.

14

Rapid Healing Foods for the Skin!

All skin diseases are merely slight variations of the same condition—inflammation of the skin caused by poisons in the body. Some are the result of taking drugs, such as arsenic, mercury, iodine, potassium, vaccines, serums, etc. Many cases are the result of bad eating habits and poor food combinations, resulting in accumulated waste in the body. Recovery hinges upon removal of the cause.

- Acne is the most common of all skin diseases and is inflammation of the oil glands of the skin and hair follicles. The first sign is usually a blackhead. Around it a pimple forms. At the tip of the pimple is a small pus-containing pustule, which hardens into a crust and falls off, leaving a small pock.

- Eczema is characterized by extreme itching. The skin is scaly and generally exudes a serum, making an additional danger of easy infection from outside bacteria. Very serious cases of infection start with eczema, poisoned by scratching bacteria into the irritated skin. The skin tends to thicken and crack, with dry patches on elbows, knees and ankles, but any area may be affected.

● **Psoriasis** is similar to eczema, but occurs mostly where there is hair growing, and there is no itching. Instead, there are raised reddish patches covered with silvery scales that peel, especially in hot weather, leaving the surface red and irritated. The hair comes out in hunks if not treated immediately. Large areas of the body may be involved, a whole leg may be covered, or it may develop only on the back, arms, elbows and ankles. It tends to get better in summer, worse in winter, may last for years, clear up suddenly, and then return.

● **Ichthyosis**, or fish skin disease, is a condition of dryness, harshness and continual scaling skin that is congenital.

There are over 100 more well-defined skin diseases. Most of them manifest themselves in the form of small pimples or eruptions. All involve inflammation, have similar causes and require similar treatment, say drugless doctors, and may be relieved quickly and completely.

THE CAUSE AND CURE
OF SKIN AILMENTS

Most skin diseases are traceable to toxic states in the inner body, rather than outside causes, say drugless doctors. As William Howard Hay, M.D. explained it, "It is not enough that the skin be kept clean in the ordinary sense, for no matter if it is washed thoroughly three times a day, scrubbed with a brush, rinsed thoroughly (with soap), it is still in far too many cases a dirty skin, because...

"...through it is continually passing all sorts of chemical debris from an internal body that is throwing off poisonous materials, which if retained would cause death in five hours or less.

"It is the passage of this internal toxic material through the skin that sets up the irritations and inflammations that we have classified and named through these many years of medical study and research. Seldom do the so-called diseases of the skin arise from outside irritations.

"As the toxic material accumulates in the body it must have an outlet or we would soon perish, and it is in seeking such an outlet that the body uses all means available, including acute fevers and colds and indigestion and chills and tonsillitis and eruptions of the covering membrane, our external organ, the skin...

"We so often see eczema, alternating with such internal conditions as neuritis or rheumatism, or asthma, and while the skin is broken out the internal condition is not in evidence, but when the skin ceases to throw off the accumulating debris then it again is manifested in the internal condition ... eczema and asthma are merely expressions of the same internal conditions, the one manifesting on the skin and the other through the bronchial tubes. *This is all that disease is, one thing, a toxic state of the entire body, and such toxic states do find expression through many and varied symptom complexes or syndromes.*

"...Every case of acne is merely an expression of an internal condition that is all wrong, and means that the lungs, skin, kidneys and bowels are among them unable to keep the body clear of its own irritating acid debris. Every boil or pimple means the same thing; every carbuncle, every eruption of whatever nature, except the few caused directly by external irritants, such as poison ivy or nettles or the bites of various insects or snakes or the application of chemical irritants directly to the skin.

"Skin allergies, by which we mean those very sensitive skins that will break out with a sort of eczema whenever brought into contact with the primrose or other vegetable irritants, are merely evidences of the internal condition of the body that makes these particular pollens irritating to these particular skins, and allergies of every sort will disappear when the body is again in proper chemical balance..."

AMAZING RELIEF CLAIMED

Acne and most other skin diseases may be remedied quickly and completely by a cleansing diet, say drugless doctors. The existing pimples will be absorbed and future eruptions will be checked. Simple acne disappears in one or two weeks, the more severe forms in a month, often permanently. Dr. Hay made these shocking claims:

● No matter what the particular skin disease, it will disappear with a cleansing diet: "Every one of the many and varied skin diseases will disappear. If you are a victim of eczema or psoriasis ... you can very easily prove this to yourself...

● "In nearly 30 years of application (of this method) I have seen no case of psoriasis or eczema that did not recover, even though both conditions had failed to improve under the most scientific treatment of many skin specialists...

● "Skin allergies ... of every sort will disappear ... in every case these allergies will disappear ... and the food that was formerly allergic may then become the favorite food and agree better than other common foods that had been the chief items of daily use."

With a cleansing diet, say drugless doctors, one may almost watch the melting away of skin diseases, and the restoration of a clean skin. Wrinkles, lines, blotches, pimples and other ugly marks vanish miraculously and leave the skin with a fine and even texture. Fine lines disappear. The scalp also gets its share of rejuvenation. Dandruff is a thing of the past and frequently new hair growth can be observed. Hardened encrustations are dissolved ... harmless tumors, cysts and congestion disappear!

DRUGLESS TREATMENT

The medical treatment for acne and other forms of skin disease consists of salves, ointments, lotions, x-rays, various drug injections and occasionally the use of vitamin A in the form of fish liver oil and synthetic vitamin B. These external applications and injections occasionally suppress the disease temporarily, but there is usually a recurrence as soon as treatment ends. These treatments often fail to provide even temporary relief, since the cause is ignored, say drugless doctors.

The drugless treatment of skin ailments consists of a short fast on water or fruit juices, cleansing the bowels, frequent bathing with plain warm water, no soap, fresh fruits and vegetables in a balanced diet, correct food combinations, avoiding starches and sugars, short sunbaths (or ultra-violet lamp treatment) and exercise to induce sweating and elimination through the skin.

Although medical doctors frequently advise against bathing, drugless doctors insist on bathing with plain warm water. Strange as it may seem, says one such doctor, that is all that is required in many cases—a few baths and the skin disease vanishes! As to sweating, "When the pores are thus opened," says Dr. Hay, "it provides an opportunity for the skin to unload freely the chemical waste matter that is carried in every body, the result of its combustion of fuel, the death of its cells and the metabolism of food materials taken in every day." The condition may appear worse for a few days, due to the increased elimination of waste matter. Bathe, keep your hands away from the area and wear light clothing.

Reported cases:

- A young man in his 20s suffered from scaly eruptions all over his body. His arms, legs, fingers, face, eyelids—even his lips—were covered with psoriasis. He had tried everything, x-rays, salves, ointments, cortisone and other drugs, to no avail. "We are doing everything we can," said his doctor. At last, he saw a drugless doctor who quickly placed him on a cleansing diet. The scaly eruptions disappeared. In a few weeks, his skin was clear. He could look in a mirror without shuddering and face the world again.

- A girl, 16, had ichthyosis (fish skin disease) which she had suffered since infancy. Although doctors say it is incurable, she recovered in six weeks with this method. Her skin returned to a normal softness and fineness with complete absence of the usual dryness, harshness and scaling.

- A doctor reports the case of a man with dark circles under his eyes. He had tried everything to get rid of them, without results. He was told to try a one-day cleansing diet. When he returned to the office, he was a different man, his face having cleared up completely. In addition, he said his dandruff disappeared and a persistent mouth condition of cracked tongue was nearly gone. "I never expected to get so much in such a short time," he said.

- "In my own case," says this doctor, "I was going bald 25 years ago and accepted it as the inevitable consequence of growing old. I was pleasantly surprised, however, to notice after (a cleansing diet) which relieved me of a serious heart condition, new hair breaking through the scalp. I have observed many similar cases, one with the restoration of a natural brunette color from a dull gray."[1]

[1]*The Natural and Drugless Way for Better Health*, by M.O. Garten (Parker Publishing Company, Inc., West Nyack, N.Y.), 1969.

FULL DETAILS ON DRUGLESS TREATMENT
FOR ACNE, ECZEMA AND PSORIASIS

A drugless osteopathic doctor reported the following cases. A boy, 16, had been suffering from severe acne for four years. The food his family ate was the usual unwholesome, greasy diet to be found in most homes. His bowels did not move oftener than every second day and, as his mother did not believe in laxatives or enemas, he continued to be constipated. His face was a mass of ugly blackheads and pimples.

"A grape fast was recommended," said this doctor, "and one of 10 days' duration was taken. The patient ate three meals a day consisting entirely of grapes without any other food, but he was under no restraint as to quantity and took as many grapes as he pleased at each meal. He drank freely of water at all times, and took two enemas per day of 1 quart each of warm water. Every other day the patient took a salt glow. He was advised to stand in the bath tub and wet the body all over, rubbing the wet skin as vigorously as possible with common salt, from the face to the feet, afterwards washing the body off with cold water, when the skin began to glow.

"The patient came to the office each day for treatment with the ultra-violet actinic ray, which was used for the face, and of such a strength as to produce a sunburn. In summertime this treatment could have been taken simply by lying in the sun with the face uncovered for 30 minutes to an hour, in which time sufficient ultra-violet rays from the sunlight could be shed upon the face to get almost as good a result as with the concentrated rays of the quartz mercury vapor lamp.

"After the fast of 10 days the patient was put on a raw food diet, taking his choice three times daily of the following uncooked foods:

Swiss chard	turnip tops	parsley
green string	kale	carrots
beans	celery	turnips
spinach	lettuce	parsnips
asparagus	cucumber	beets
oyster plant		
beet tops		

"These foods were combined together in different ways to suit the taste of the patient, and no other food of any kind was used for about 15 days. Large quantities of water were also drunk with this diet.

"Before the end of the raw food diet the face was entirely cleared of any sign of acne or pimples. After the 15 days of raw food diet the patient was put on a general diet regime and was warned against too free a use of fatty foods and sugar. At the time of writing, after an interval of more than three years, the patient has had no return of the trouble."

***

An eight-year-old boy suffered with eczema since a few days after birth. He'd been treated by many doctors, and many patent medicines and salves had been used with absolutely no effect. Doctors said they never saw a more stubborn case.

He was finally brought to this drugless doctor, who recalled: "A water fast was used for four days. Three times daily a teaspoonful of common baking soda was added to the water, so that the boy had what might be called an alkaline water fast. At the end of that time all itching had disappeared, and the skin was almost entirely clear. The child was put on a well-balanced diet, avoiding antagonistic mixtures of food, but using almost every kind of food in season, and in perfectly proportioned combinations. This cure was effected over six years ago, and there has been no return of any symptom of eczema since that time.

***

A man, 35, had been suffering with psoriasis since early childhood, and lost all his body hair, on account of it. At this time, the disease was extending rapidly through the hair on his head. The hair was trimmed short, and ultra-violet light—which can be obtained from the sun—was used on the scalp. A straight water fast was used for a month, and at the end of that time the skin was almost entirely clear.

"The patient was a small man weighing 125 pounds and worked constantly during the fast in a machine shop, doing hard manual labor," said this doctor. "He now has a luxuriant growth of hair, without any sign of a return of any skin disease. He now eats almost anything he wants, and has remained cured for over four years."

RAPID HEALING FOODS FOR THE SKIN

Athlete's foot can be cured by garlic. The method is to spread some freshly crushed garlic over the area. It will feel warm for about five minutes. After a half hour, wash with plain water. Do this once a day for a week, and goodbye athlete's foot. (If the skin burns, wash immediately with plain water and try later with less garlic.) To prevent reinfection boil your stockings.

Bedsores can be healed with soybean lecithin. A nurse reports using ordinary liquid lecithin—purchased at a local health food store—to heal two bedsores on the lower spine of a gentleman patient at the hospital where she worked. Three times a day the sores were cleaned with hydrogen peroxide, coated with liquid lecithin, and bandaged with non-stick dressing. The man did not lean on the sores. In two days, everyone was surprised to find the bedsores healing. Garlic can heal bedsores. A man suffering bedsores had tried everything else for a year without success, when he read that garlic was good for boils and suppurating sores. He diced some garlic in tiny bits, mixed it with oil and made a poultice. It burned, but he left it on for two days. When he took off the pad, he couldn't believe his eyes. The scab was off, the swelling was down, no bleeding. After this he applied a comfrey salve, and it was all smooth in a week.

Blisters can be healed with garlic oil. A letter carrier with painful blisters tried every medicine on the market with absolutely no results. Then he remembered the antiseptic properties of garlic. He spread some garlic oil on his blistered feet, and the swelling vanished overnight, with no more pain. His doctor was amazed.

Boils can be relieved with garlic mixed with oil or lard. Garlic kills the staphylococci germs in boils and heals all manner of suppurating (running) sores.

Burns can be healed with apple cider vinegar. A man whose shirt caught fire from flaming gasoline screamed for help. A neighbor ripped off his shirt and poured apple cider vinegar on his back. He said the pain was immediately gone. It never returned and there were no scars. Many others report the same amazing relief. Honey can bring spectacular relief from burns. One man who was horribly scalded from head to foot by boiling water, with terrible pain that nearly drove him mad, got immediate relief with honey. His wife and daughter dabbed it all over his body. Instantly the pain stopped, he slept all night, and didn't lose a single hair. His doctor couldn't believe it.

Carbuncles vanish with honey. One man had two large carbuncles on his back. One was operated on by a surgeon and left a deep, ugly scar. The other he treated with honey. Although enormous in size, the second carbuncle rapidly disappeared, leaving only a tiny dot.

Cold sores can be relieved with sage tea. A very old and simple remedy that really works is to make a cup of sage tea (two or three leaves per cup). When steeped, add 1 teaspoon of powdered ginger. It relieves a sore mouth and upset stomach. One user reports her cold sores disappeared after three cups of tea. Another time she tried it, and they disappeared overnight.

Diabetic dent marks may be cured with peanut oil. This is an ailment in which insulin causes flesh to disappear at the site of injections, creating "dents" or "craters" ranging in size from very small dimples to large, deep holes. One woman who had this was told there was no cure, but accidentally discovered that peanut oil made the dents smooth out. Taking care never to touch or press inside them, she applied more oil every day. She also found that by gaining a few pounds—keeping them on a couple of months—and then losing them, the dents filled in faster. In two years, most of the dents all over her body disappeared.

Eczema can be healed with blackstrap molasses. One user reports that 2 teaspoons of blackstrap molasses taken in a glass of milk twice daily cured it. Another reports that after seven years, and numerous visits to a doctor, during which nothing helped, this method cured her. In two weeks, her skin was almost 100 percent normal. Brewer's yeast can heal eczema. A woman with severe eczema on her hands, with scales, red bumps, cracks, itching and swelling, discovered that taking brewer's yeast (6 tablets a day) for a few days, cleared it up completely. Raw potatoes can cure eczema and other skin eruptions. A girl who had suffered severe eczema since childhood, was spending $25 a week for drugstore medications—which gave temporary relief—when an older woman advised her to eat raw potatoes. She stopped taking drugs, and after a few weeks on the raw potato diet, her face cleared up. She continues to eat one daily.

Erysipelas can be healed with honey. It is said that an amazingly effective remedy is to cover the area—and a little beyond—with lots of honey, dress with cotton, and allow to remain for 24 hours, repeating as necessary.

Fatty tumors and sebaceous cysts may be healed with soybean lecithin. One woman who kept getting fatty growths inside her body that cut off circulation near her lungs and heart, had to have surgery several times. Then she started taking lecithin and vitamin C. Since then, a growth in her ankle, and a lump between two ribs (sebaceous cyst) have almost vanished.

Fingernails that are brittle or peeling can be strengthened by eating sunflower seeds. People with such problems claim that eating sunflower seeds every day makes the nails hard and strong.

Gangrene may be cured with honey. An elderly woman was admitted to a hospital with gangrene of the foot. Doctors wanted to amputate, but decided she could not survive an operation. Instead, her foot was covered with honey. It healed and she walked away completely cured. A diabetic woman was suffering from a horrible foot infection, was in excruciating pain and could hardly walk. Doctors had removed one toe, and wanted to amputate the rest of the foot. Then she heard how diabetics can avoid amputation due to early hardening of the arteries and bad circulation in the legs by soaking them in warm salt water, or peroxide and water. To her doctor's amazement, in a week it was almost completely healed, pain and swelling were gone, no amputation was needed, and she was pronounced cured. A 30-year-old man had gangrene patches on the fingers of one hand. Using 500 mg of vitamin E and nothing else except vitamin E ointment, the hideous purple patches changed to normal pink tissue, and healed completely in two months.

Impetigo can be cured with garlic oil. Standard medical treatment can take two weeks, with sticky medication, and unbearable itching. By spreading garlic oil on the irritated areas, one user reports, in a half hour the itching was gone completely, and she was able to sleep all night. In three days, the condition seemed to vanish altogether.

Infections can be relieved by onion. One woman had an agonizing infection from a sliver of wood under her fingernail. It was impossible to remove, and the finger was badly swollen and painful. She took a slice of onion and taped it around the area and overnight, swelling, plus sliver, had disappeared completely.

Leg ulcers from varicose veins can be healed with honey. Usually, these do not heal easily, particularly in the elderly, but it is said that regular daily application of honey can soon reduce the infection and bring about a complete healing. Okra can heal leg ulcers, too. A man with diabetes was suffering from a leg ulcer that would not heal. Cortisone and other antibiotic ointments failed. Finally, he tried placing a fresh clean okra leaf on the ulcer, three times a day. This healed it where all else failed. Total time: about a month. Comfrey can heal stubborn ulcers, burns and open wounds with spectacular results. A man with varicose leg ulcers failed to get relief after two years of ointments and bandages—recommended by a doctor. A friend advised him to try a poultice of comfrey leaves once a day. In a little over a month, the ulcers healed completely. An elderly man suddenly developed a large fulminating ulcer on his foot. It spread rapidly, exposing the bones. His condition looked hopeless until his daughter decided to apply dressings soaked in comfrey tea, every four hours. The ulcer immediately began to fill up rapidly and was almost completely healed in a month. A woman with a large gangrenous ulcer full of pus on her leg faced amputation. Comfrey was applied in dressings. In a week, islands of healing appeared. In three weeks, this huge ulcer was reduced to the size of a pinhead.

Liver spots have disappeared with the addition of 100 mg of vitamin E to every meal. Brown liver spots all over the arms of women who have passed menopause, and large irregular brown spots on the face as big as ¾ of an inch have faded away and completely disappeared, in as little as six weeks. Wrinkles seem to smooth out and melt away with large doses of this rapid healing food.

Poison ivy can be healed by lemon juice. One man accidentally sat in some poison ivy. His entire body broke out in a massive inflammation, with itching that could only be relieved by soaking in a tub. A doctor's ointment gave him "cortisone bumps" on his fingers and made it worse. Then he remembered reading that lemon juice can help many skin conditions, including acne, eczema, erysipelas, boils, carbuncles, blackheads, dandruff, insect bites and poison oak and ivy. He sliced open a couple of lemons and rubbed them all over his body. In less than 5 minutes, his skin looked completely normal, and he felt immediate relief. (An orange works as well.)

Poison oak can be healed by goldenseal. A woman with a severe case of poison oak, covering her entire body, including eyes and ears, suffered three weeks of sleepless nights and agony, before discovering this remedy. She drank some golden-seal tea (½ teaspoon per cup). In 20 minutes the itching stopped. Then she made a wash (1 teaspoon to a pint of hot water), and the healing could be seen immediately.

Psoriasis can be healed by soybean lecithin. People with red, itching and even bleeding scales on their elbows, people who had tried all kinds of creams and medications to no avail, long-time sufferers with psoriasis from head to foot, claim that all scaling has completely disappeared since using lecithin.

Stings can be relieved with wheat germ oil, honey or raw sliced onion. One lady got a yellow jacket sting between two toes. By the time she got home, her foot was three times its normal size. She applied some raw sliced onion to it. In less than 30 minutes, her foot was back to normal, and never knew it had been stung. A man was mowing his lawn, dressed in shorts, when a swarm of hornets attacked him. He dashed into the house and rolled on the floor to dislodge some hornets that were still biting him, and screamed for a doctor. His wife dabbed honey all over his legs and arms. His terrible pains were relieved almost immediately, with hardly any swelling. Wheat germ oil relieves stings. Users say that hornet stings have been relieved immediately, with no swelling.

Vitiligo (white patches on skin) has been cured with pure mayonnaise. One woman says this has worked for her, and all others who've tried it, after doctors had told her it was incurable. She claims it restores the acid mantle of the skin which soap and detergents destroy. In one week, the color began returning to her skin. In severe cases, it may take several months, but it works, she says. In another case, a woman with vitiligo who lost all the pigmentation of her skin on her entire body, cured herself with massive doses of B vitamins. It also made excruciating burning sensations in her shoulder (whenever she lifted something) disappear.

Warts and growths can be removed with cabbage juice, comfrey or garlic. One woman with hundreds of ugly black warts all over her face, neck and chest was advised to drink lots of raw cabbage juice. In a few weeks, the ugly mess cleared up entirely. An elderly woman had an ugly, red, nipple-shaped growth on her nose, which kept growing back even when removed, sur-gically. Finally, she applied comfrey root poultices day and night. Almost immediately, the inflammation was gone, and the wart soon disappeared. Garlic oil can remove harmless growths.

A dentist reports that for 10 years he underwent x-ray and radium treatments to eradicate ugly skin growths that kept reappearing, even though a doctor said they were non-malignant. On applying garlic oil, the painful growths on his face, some of them enormous, disappeared in about a month. Garlic can make warts disappear overnight in many cases. Pimples disappear without a trace if rubbed several times a day with garlic.

QUICK RUNDOWN OF FOODS THAT HAVE BEEN USED IN TREATING SPECIFIC AILMENTS

Starred items refer to use as external dressing or for external application only. Otherwise the food should be eaten. Two stars mean the food may be eaten or used as a dressing or both.

Acne

asparagus
beets
beet tops
carrots
celery
cucumber
grapes
green string
  beans
kale
lemon juice
lettuce
oyster plant
parsley
parsnips
spinach
sunbaths
Swiss chard
turnips
turnip tops
water

Antiseptic for Wounds

**lemon juice

Athlete's Foot

*garlic crushed

Baldness

**garlic
**onion
squash
sunflower
  seeds

Bedsores

*soybean
  lecithin
  liquid
*garlic, diced

Blackheads

*lemon juice

Blisters

*garlic oil

Burns

*apple cider
  vinegar

*banana
*cocoanut oil
*comfrey leaves
  or tea
honey
*olive oil
  (sunburns)
*potato, raw,
  crushed

Boils, Carbuncles

*aloe vera (liquid from
  leaf)
*banana
*garlic mixed
  with lard or
  oil
*honey
  (carbuncles)
*lemon (small
  boiled slice)
*onion, crushed
*potato, raw,
  crushed

Chickenpox

honey

Clogged Pores

*mango

Cold Sores

sage tea (2-3
  leaves per
  cup, plus one
  teaspoon
  powdered
  ginger, 3
  cups daily)

Cuts

*cocoanut oil

Cysts

*mango

Dandruff

*lemon juice
*yucca plant
  shampoo

*Diabetic Dent
  Marks*

*Peanut oil (ap-
  plied around
  dents, never
  inside, plus
  gaining a
  few pounds,
  holding the
  gain for two
  months and
  losing it—re-
  peated over a
  period of
  time)

Dry Skin

squash
sunflower
  seeds
vitamin A
vitamin B
  complex
linoleic acid

Eczema

beet juice
black currant
  juice
blackstrap
  molasses (2
  teaspoons in
  a glass of
  milk twice
  daily)
carrot juice
**cucumber
lemon juice
nettle juice
potatoes, raw
water fast (3
  days)

Erysipelas

*honey
*lemon juice

*Fatty Tumors
  and
  Sebaceous
  Cysts*

soybean
  lecithin
vitamin C

Fingernails

sunflower
  seeds

Freckles

*lemon juice

Gangrene

*honey dressing
*warm salt
  water
*peroxide and
  water
**vitamin E

Impetigo

*garlic oil

Leg Ulcers

apple juice
*cabbage leaves
citrus juices
*comfrey
  leaves, tea
*goldenseal,
  mashed
*honey
*okra leaf
onion and
  garlic juice
  added to
  carrot juice
*papaya leaves
*yellow onion

Pimples

apricots
*comfrey salve
cranberries
tomatoes (in
  large
  quantity)

Poison Ivy

Brewer's yeast (large doses with warm water and honey throughout the day)
**goldenseal tea (½ teaspoon per cup, or as wash 1 teaspoon to pint of water)

Psoriasis

soybean lecithin

Pyorrhea

*lemon rind applied to gums

Ringworm

*strawberries, crushed
*tomatoes

Skin Eruptions

*olive oil
pears
plums
potatoes, raw, 1 daily
tangerines

Skin Infections

*garlic mixed with oil or lard
*lemon juice
*wheat germ oil

Vitiligo

*pure mayonnaise

vitamin B complex

Warts and Growths

cabbage juice
*castor oil
*comfrey root
*garlic oil

Wrinkles

*cocoanut oil (apply after lemon juice)
*lemon juice (allow to dry and remove with olive oil after a few hours)
*olive oil

15

=

Rapid Healing Foods
for Arthritis!

–

Practically all forms of arthritis can be speedily remedied, with rapid healing foods—say drugless doctors. For many years it was thought, even by drugless doctors, that ankylosed (or fused) joints and deformities could not be corrected, but there is now startling evidence that even these can be restored, without surgery, in many cases.

Medical doctors say there is no known cause or cure for arthritis. They *think* the basic cause is infection of some sort, starting at a certain focal point, and lodging in the joints. In the hope of remedying the arthritis, surgery is often used. The sinuses are scraped, teeth, tonsils, even bones and joints are removed. Drugs are used to kill pain, fight infection, relieve swelling. Artificial joints are inserted. Painful exercises are recommended to keep the patient "limber."

There is much continued suffering, as anyone who has gone the drug route will notice—and this state of affairs has not changed much in 50 years. Bony overgrowth continues to form, in many cases *even over artificial joints*. With that in mind, here is the drugless system, which medical doctors say is nonsense.

THE CAUSE AND CURE OF ARTHRITIS

Arthritics will continue to suffer, as long as the *cause* is ignored, say drugless doctors. We know the cause and cure right now, they say. We've known it for at least 50 years. And all the medicine and surgery in the world will not cure arthritis, if—by our eating habits—we continue to cause it.

Fundamentally and primarily the cause of arthritis is toxemia—an overloading of poisons—the result of heavy eating, especially of sweets and starches, bread, potatoes, cakes, pies and candy, drinking, wrong food combinations, nervous tension, sexual overindulgence and physical overactivity, say drugless doctors.

Any one of these habits can cause a build-up of poisons—too numerous to uncover and label by name. It is not necessary to waste years trying to isolate each one, while millions suffer, when we know how to get rid of them *now*, say drugless doctors. In light of recent research, arthritis may be caused by a hormonal imbalance, by infections, by any of a thousand different chemical disturbances. For those who like explanations, the basic theory of toxemia (internal poisoning) was explained this way by a drugless osteopathic doctor:

"One of the principal causes of rheumatism is toxemia produced from the fermentation of an excess of carbohydrate foods, or from poison generated by fermentation when these foods are used in wrong combination. In the treatment of any form of (arthritis) the use of the fasting cure will be found to be the means of getting the quickest results possible...

"The bloodstream during the fasting period cleanses itself from all of these toxins which set up irritation in the muscles or joints, or in the nerve trunks, and are thus responsible for every form of rheumatic disorder ... usually the muscular soreness will leave in two or three days after beginning the fast ... You may expect the permanent cure to take at least as long as it would take a broken bone to heal."

Another drugless doctor, an M.D. who abandoned drugs after his own health failed and has recovered without them, stated:

"Arthritis represents such an imbalance in the chemistry of the body, such an acid-alkali imbalance, that waste matter is cast out of the circulation into those regions where the bloodstream is slowest, as the fibrous tissues about the joints...

"Aside from (a) daily or twice daily toilette of the colon, arthritis needs only the very same dietary care as is necessary for health in anyone, merely a discontinuance of all the causes of disease as these arise from the digestive tract, as is shown by the body's inability to carry incalculable amounts of chemical debris without spilling it somewhere."

And again, we are told by one of the great exponents of a cleansing diet and rapid cleansing foods:

"Nothing can more certainly or more rapidly alter the state of the nutrition of the body than a fast. No other means at our disposal brings about a more rapid change in the chemistry of the body ... Fasting relieves the pains of arthritis, for example, more effectively than drugs and does it without risk or harm."

Fasting or some form of cleansing diet has always been used by drugless doctors, with the best success, in clearing up arthritis. In almost every case, pain, swelling and inflammation vanish in a remarkably short time, joints that were rigid and immovable become free and flexible, even in advanced cases.

EASY CLEANSING DIETS TO RELIEVE ARTHRITIC PAINS

While methods may vary slightly, among drugless doctors, the basic principles remain the same: remove the causes, drain the body of its poisons, feed it properly and miracles of healing happen. One drugless doctor, an osteopathic physician, reported the following cases:

"A 54-year-old man came to me suffering from rheumatism in the left shoulder. Several doctors had told him he would never be able to raise his arm again sufficiently to be able to work at his occupation as a rancher. Because of the fact that all efforts to cure the rheumatism in the shoulder failed, the last doctors he consulted

advised him to stop using his arm entirely, and allow the bones of the shoulder to grow together...

"The patient was immediately started on a fast of water and lemon juice, drinking at least one glass of water every 30 minutes all during the day. He was advised to add to each glass the juice of half a lemon ... By the tenth day of the fast, without any treatment being applied to the shoulder, he had sufficiently recovered to be able to work eight hours a day picking lemons. In picking lemons ... it is necessary ... to hold the hand at least a foot above the shoulder. This he was able to do without any apparent discomfort beyond the fact that his arm was weak from long disuse ... after the tenth day of the fast no pain whatever was present.

"The fast was, however, continued for 10 days more, after which the patient was put upon a well-regulated diet, and has continued to be well for over seven years, with no sign of a return of any form of rheumatism."

AN AMAZING RECOVERY

This same doctor stated: "A woman, 45, had suffered from rheumatism all her life, and by the time I was called in on her case she had been confined to the house for over 10 years, for weeks at a time being unable to leave her bed. The disease had reached the stage of arthritis deformans, and the fingers were twisted out of shape, with very little movement to the elbows and shoulders. The ankles were swollen to about twice their normal size, and a great deal of bone change had taken place, greatly enlarging the joints.

"She immediately started upon a fast, using the juice of one orange every two hours, together with a glass of water. She was also advised to take a glass of water every 15 minutes during her waking hours, and as she was unable to come to the office for treatment, no local treatments of any kind were given except bathing the feet in hot epsom-salt water and having a hot-water bottle constantly at her feet (this will keep the circulation almost as good as if the patient were exercising, and still there will be no irritation of the joints). Two enemas daily were taken.

"At the end of one week of this fast the swelling had reduced so materially in the ankles, with a corresponding decrease of soreness, that she was able to walk three blocks to a street car and ride several miles to my office ... This was the first time she had been able to come downtown for over 10 years. From that time on she improved rapidly..."

The doctor stated that her fast was continued for 21 days, and then she was put on the following: ¼ pound Salisbury steak, with either raw tomatoes or celery, four times daily (30 minutes before and after each meal, a half pint of hot water was to be taken, and as much water as possible at other times). Two enemas daily were prescribed, to ensure a free cleansing of the bowels. After two months, she resumed a general diet. In the years since, we are told, she never had a return of any rheumatic pain, feels quite well, and is able to do her own housework!

UNLOCKING FROZEN JOINTS

In both these cases, we have seen the actual unlocking of frozen joints. On a cleansing diet, free motion is easily restored to joints that are rigid and nearly immovaole. Enlarged joints are considerably reduced in size and made movable once again— all without drugs or surgery. Relief has been noted in thousands of cases. In *The Natural and Drugless Way for Better Health* (Parker Publishing Company, Inc., 1969), M.O. Garten, D.C. says:

> **"One of my patients, a lady of 62, was suffering from arthritis in both knees. The joints were greatly enlarged and for the past 12 years the patient had tried frantically to get relief from the stiffness and excruciating pains. Every type of treatment had been tried and had failed. The patient was finally put on a fast, and ... according to her report the pain left her on the ninth day. (Three weeks later) I found the lady in tears of joy— she discovered she was now able to do knee bends."**

"I have seen many patients that had typical arthritic hands where the knuckle joints were enlarged, sometimes even deformed. On a complete water fast (a cleansing diet), increased motion was experienced by these patients after the seventh day," says Dr. Garten. On a cleansing diet, he points out, waste material—including waste material in bones and joints—is dissolved and excreted.

A DOCTOR'S PROVEN NEW HOME CURE
FOR ARTHRITIS

But what if the bones are actually fused? For a long time, drugless doctors freely admitted that in advanced cases this could not be reversed. It remained for Giraud W. Campbell, D.O., to discover how this could be done, as revealed in his book, *A Doctor's Proven New Home Cure for Arthritis* (Parker Publishing Company, Inc., 1972).

Dr. Campbell says his method has cured hundreds of sufferers, regardless of age or condition. In all cases, heat and swelling in the affected joints was eased within one week. Pain was relieved, in most cases eliminated, in two weeks or less. Normal movement was restored in almost all cases in three weeks or less. X-rays revealed progress in the restoration of damaged bone structure in three to six months.

Wheelchairs and crutches were tossed aside. The only cases to whom he cannot guarantee relief, he says, are those who have had extensive gold or drug therapy (which sometimes permanently alters the body chemistry), and advanced spinal arthritis if not caught within the first five years. Even so, spectacular relief is reported in many such cases, and further bone degeneration is halted. Even the agony of weather changes can be a thing of the past, he says.

Not only are pain and inflammation relieved, bone structure is improved, says Dr. Campbell, offering x-rays that show kneecaps unfusing, compressed vertebrae regenerating, bony overgrowth reduced and absorbed—which medical doctors consider impossible. "Those that are bed-ridden ... in the acute inflammatory state ... show the most dramatic response," he says. "In from three to 10 days their pains cease, and repair sets in."

Dr. Campbell gives the following cases:

- **A woman said: "I found myself a cripple, unable to walk without pain. I tried several doctors, aspirin, gold injections, cortisone drugs—nothing seemed to help. I kept**

getting continually worse, endured constant pain and had
to be pulled from a chair, helped at every step." After four
years of suffering, she tried this method and says: "Within
three weeks I was without pain and could go to work
feeling my old self again ... jump out of bed and feel alive. I
am now able to stand up straight, move about without
pain, get a good night's sleep and do housework. I enjoy
life again."

• Mrs. A.S., 65, began to experience pains and stiffness in
her arms and legs. Her doctor called it arthritis (rheumatoid) and treated her for one month. Then he sent her to
a specialist, who referred her to another specialist, who
gave her six months of treatment and sent her to a medical
center for cobalt treatment (another six months). No cure,
they all said. With this method, she said: "I am able to arise
in the morning, make my own bed, walk up and down
stairs, go out to dine, visit friends and go shopping..."

• Walter M. said: "I was in agony. Something was wrong with
my spine in the region of my shoulder blades. I had visited
medical men ... and I could not obtain relief. The neuro-
surgeon prescribed traction ... which did not ease my pain
... I could not sleep in bed ... I had to sleep in an upright
position at the dining room table." With this method, in two
weeks he could once again sleep in comfort.

• Mrs. G.W., 42, was in such pain she could not stand the
pressure of bedsheets, and she'd been bedridden six
months. Even her jaw was painful. With this method in two
days her pain was gone, without medication or aspirin. In
two weeks she was walking and housecleaning. Her hands
no longer bothered her. After six months, you'd never
guess she had arthritis.

• One man said shortly after his Army service, he began
experiencing pain in his lower back and shooting pains
down the back of his legs. Doctors gave him no relief. He
could hardly move and was in constant agony. He spent
four years, going to a VA hospital, with no relief. Then he
tried an arthritic specialist for *nine years*, with all kinds of
medications and injections. He grew steadily worse. His
spine practically fused solid. Then he heard about this
method of rapid healing foods. In two weeks, 50 percent of
his pain vanished. He was able to walk better, and gradually straightened up. Years of agony vanished!

"Arthritis can be cured," says Dr. Campbell. "While a search for a cure for arthritis goes on, *hundreds, for a fact, are being cured,"* he emphasizes. "While scientists theorize about the high white blood cell count or the low red blood cell count, hundreds of arthritic sufferers are emerging from their ordeal with a normal blood count. While scientists are debating over bacteria, viruses and mycoplasma, the disease is abating (with this method) ... While new salicylates, like aspirin, are perfected to relieve those whose lives are destined to be plagued by arthritic pain, that *pain is gone forever within seven days for those who eat in a special way* ... While patients are being injected with (drugs), with ACTH and with gold ... others are injecting themselves with delicious nutritional foods and enjoying *permanent cure* ... (with) no need for aspirin or other pain relievers in a week or 10 days ... a gradual restoration of damaged bone ... return to a normal life without arthritic pain."

SEVEN-DAY PROGRAM TO END ARTHRITIC PAIN AND REGAIN NORMAL USE OF JOINTS

The cause of arthritis, says Dr. Campbell, is devitalized food—fast food items—that cause nutritional deficiency and pollution. After years of irritation, arthritic sufferers become allergic to these foods, he says. These include prepared and processed foods, packaged desserts, canned foods, ice cream, cake and candy. All these sugar and chemical-laden foods are poison, he says. The foods that cure arthritis are fresh fruits, garden fresh vegetables, fish and certain meats. Dr. Campbell says the following diet will relieve all types of arthritis, including osteoarthritis, rheumatoid arthritis or any other type of arthritis.

Day No. 1

Breakfast—none
Lunch—   none
Dinner— none

Stay away from food completely for one full day. Drink at least four 8-ounce glasses of water.

Day No. 2

Breakfast—Unsweetened grape or prune juice.
　　　　　Bananas.
Lunch—　　Fresh beef liver, preferably raw or lightly
　　　　　sauteed.
　　　　　Mixed green salad, oil and vinegar dressing.
　　　　　Bowl of blueberries or other fruit in season.
Dinner—　 Raw vegetable plate (green peppers, celery,
　　　　　tomatoes, etc.).
　　　　　Raw fruit salad (shred apples, figs, grapes, ba-
　　　　　nanas, etc., but no citrus fruits).

Take 1 tablespoon of cod liver oil, twice a day.

Day No. 3

Breakfast—Blended raw fruits.
　　　　　8 oz. raw certified milk.
Lunch—　　Fresh filet of ocean fish lightly sauteed.
　　　　　Raw cauliflower or other raw fresh vegetable.
　　　　　8 oz. certified milk with 1 tablespoon of powdered
　　　　　brewer's yeast and 1 tablespoon of blackstrap
　　　　　molasses.
Dinner—　 Fresh (or kosher) beef liver lightly sauteed with
　　　　　onions.
　　　　　Mixed green salad.
　　　　　Melon, or other fruit in season.
　　　　　8 oz. raw certified milk.

Take 1 tablespoon of cod liver oil, twice a day.

Day No. 4

Breakfast—Prunes or prune juice.
　　　　　8 oz. raw certified milk.
Lunch—　　Veal kidneys, lightly sauteed.
　　　　　Mixed green salad.
　　　　　8 oz. raw certified milk with 1 tablespoon powdered
　　　　　brewer's yeast and 1 tablespoon of blackstrap
　　　　　molasses.
Dinner—　 Halibut steak (or other seafood) broiled.
　　　　　Raw spinach salad.
　　　　　Half avocado.
　　　　　Strawberries or other fruit in season.
　　　　　8 oz. raw certified milk.

Take 1 tablespoon of cod liver oil, twice a day.

Day No. 5

Breakfast—Cantaloupe half, or other raw fruit in season.
8 oz. raw certified milk.

Lunch— Half avocado, sliced tomatoes and watercress.
8 oz. raw certified milk with 1 tablespoon of powdered brewer's yeast and 1 tablespoon of blackstrap molasses.

Dinner— Fresh beef liver patties, as rare as you can eat them.
Mixed green salad.
Rhubarb.
8 oz. raw certified milk.

Take 1 tablespoon cod liver oil, twice a day.

Day No. 6

Breakfast—Unsweetened grape or prune juice.
Veal kidneys lightly sauteed.
8 ozs. raw certified milk

Lunch— Shrimp salad.
Cantaloupe half, or other raw fruit in season.
8 oz. raw certified milk with 1 tablespoon of powdered brewer's yeast and 1 tablespoon of blackstrap molasses.

Dinner— Large chef's salad including raw peas, raw string beans, and other uncooked vegetables and greens.
Plums or other raw fruit in season.
8 oz. raw certified milk.

Take 1 tablespoon of cod liver oil, twice a day.

Day No. 7

Breakfast—Sliced bananas.
8 oz. raw certified milk.

Lunch— Lightly broiled filet of sole.
Carrot sticks and watercress.
Grapes.
8 oz. raw certified milk.

Dinner— Lightly sauteed sweetbreads.
Raw vegetables mixed in blender.
Honeydew melon or other raw fruit in season.
8 oz. raw certified milk.

Take 1 tablespoon of cod liver oil, twice a day.

Many facets of this program have been known and used for many years by drugless healers. Fasting, for example, internal cleansing (enemas, see below), fresh fruits and vegetables, cod liver oil. It took Dr. Campbell to put it all together, for the first time, in his proven new home cure for arthritis. During all seven days:

1. Drink only when thirsty, and then only raw fresh fruit or raw fresh vegetable juice, or raw certified milk or water.

2. Take an enema daily until charcoal or corn test show no further need. (Purchase charcoal tablets at health food store. Take six at the end of an evening meal. They color your stool black. The entire black should be eliminated the following morning. In arthritis, it usually takes from four days to a week for the black to disappear. The next night instead of charcoal eat one or two ears of corn for dinner. Swallow some of the kernels whole. The following day, these should appear in the stool. If not, take a warm-water enema.)

3. Continue this diet until heat, pain and swelling disappear.

4. Add one food per day after heat, pain and swelling disappear, from the allowable lists.

ALLOWABLE FOODS

Vegetables

carrots
peas
black-eyed peas
green peppers
lima beans
string beans
pole beans
wax beans
navy beans
corn
cucumbers
hubbard squash
golden squash
butternut squash
banana squash
zucchini squash
summer squash
red cabbage
savoy cabbage

spinach
kale
Swiss chard
kohlrabi
tomatoes
beet tops
radishes
parsnips
cauliflower
rutabagas
turnips
eggplant
broccoli
Brussels sprouts
parsley
salsify
asparagus
onions
scallions
leeks
chives

okra
mushrooms
horseradish
brown rice
wild rice
lettuce
watercress
endive
escarole
beets

Fruits

golden apples
red apples
Northern spry
   apples
Rome apples
Baldwin apples
russets
winesaps
Cortlands

bananas
sickel pears
blueberries
raspberries
strawberries
gooseberries
loganberries
mulberries
rhubarb
currants
figs
prunes
plums
nectarines
peaches
Bartlett pears
boysenberries
apricots
cherries
grapes (all
 varieties)
melons (all
 varieties)

Nuts

hazel nuts
walnuts
Brazil nuts
almonds
pecans
peanuts
Chinese
 chestnuts
butternuts
filberts
black walnuts
hickory nuts
cashews

Seeds

pumpkin
sunflower
sesame

Fowl

range chicken
duck
goose
turkey
Cornish hen
squab

Meats (beef)

roasts (all kinds)
shank meat
chopped beef
stew beef
steaks (all kinds)
short ribs
flanken
ox tails

Meats (lambs)

roast leg of lamb
lamb shank
chops (all kinds)
lamb patties
lamb stew

Meats (pork)

roasts (all kinds)
chops (all kinds)
sausage
 (homemade)
head cheese
pigs knuckles
spareribs

Meats (veal)

chops
cutlets (not
 breaded)
veal roast
breast of veal

Meats (organ)

liver
kidney
heart
brains
sweetbreads
tripe (cattle only)

Seafood

striped bass
cod
flounder
halibut
tuna (fresh)
whiting
scallops (bay)
scallops (deep
 sea)
lobster
shrimp
crabs (soft)
crabs (hard)
red snapper
eels
pompano
sea bass
fluke
smelts
salmon (fresh)
clams
mussels
oysters
concha
shad (boned)
fish roe

Soups

split pea soup
lentil
marrowbone
lima bean
barley
 (unpearled)
navy bean

FOODS TO BE PERMANENTLY AVOIDED

1. Flour of all kinds, whether it is whole wheat (unless grown without artificial fertilizers and poisonous sprays), white flour, corn flour, rye flour, soy flour, etc.
2. All flour products, like bread, toasts, cakes, pies, cookies, crackers, buns, crullers, doughnuts, spaghetti, macaroni, noodles, pizza, etc.
3. Coffee, tea, cocoa, liquor, beer, wine, colas, carbonated beverages and all so-called "soft drinks."
4. Sugars, candies, ice cream and artificial sweeteners.
5. Jellies, jams and marmalades.
6. Canned or processed foods such as jello, custard, pudding and prepared mixes.
7. Frozen fruits.
8. Any food manufactured or adulterated by man, such as: prepared breakfast cereals or semi-prepared ones like quick-cooked oatmeal.

You may be able to cheat, from time to time, and get away with it. But you should always be on your guard for adverse symptoms or flareups, and immediately go back to this program, says Dr. Campbell.

In Dr. Campbell's list of allowed foods, you'll notice you get your B vitamins from liver, Brewer's yeast and blackstrap molasses (iron, too); you get your calcium from fresh vegetables; your A and D vitamins from cod liver oil and your iodine from fish. In his book, *An Eighty-Year-Old Doctor's Secrets of Positive Health*, William Brady, M.D. states: "If you ask me about 'rheumatiz' (that's what he calls all forms of arthritis), I'll tell you it is a degeneration of the joint tissues due to nutritional deficiency.. and that *it is chiefly a calcium, vitamin D, iodine and vitamin B deficiency. There is no more to tell about the nature and cause of insidiously developing joint disability of long standing* ...

"This is not something I picked out of the air. It is a conviction that came from a professional lifetime of study ... I am not promoting any remedy or cure. I merely recommend a regimen, a way of life to prevent, relieve...perhaps even cure the 'rheumatiz.' This last claim I hesitate to make. But I am emboldened to speak of cure by numerous reports I have received from victims who declare they really are cured and back at their jobs."

The main difference between Brady's program and Campbell's is that Brady, an M.D., ignores most food sources of these nutrients (he does recommend 1½ pints of milk, cod liver oil and plain wheat daily). He suggests you get your calcium, vitamins D, B-complex and iodine from high-potency tablets, at your local health food store. He makes no mention of what foods to avoid, or internal cleansing. While users no longer required aspirin or pain relievers, after 10 days, there is no real difference between being chained to one type of pill or another, an aspirin or a calcium tablet. Except for the fact that if you can't stand the taste of cod liver oil, Dr. Campbell says it's okay to use a capsule, and he does recommend Brewer's yeast (a concentrated protein), Campbell's program uses only food as medicine.

Cod liver oil has been known to relieve arthritis for 50 years, ever since Dr. Ralph Pemberton used it to treat 400 arthritic patients, most of whom were helped. This was reported in the *Archives of Internal Medicine* (March 1920). Dr. Pemberton's method was essentially controlled fasting in which certain foods were allowed, but patients were kept away from starches, sugar and flour.

Medical doctors are slowly starting to realize the value of these methods. In an article in the *Journal of the National Medical Association*, Charles A. Brusch, M.D. and Edward T. Johnson, M.D. obtained rapid and astonishing results in relieving arthritis and rheumatism, with a partial fasting or cleansing diet. The main points of this plan are the taking of cod liver oil on an empty stomach and the restriction of all water intake to a single portion taken one hour before breakfast.

As reported by Carlson Wade,[1] these doctors tested 98 patients, and found 92 showed major improvement in their arthritic symptoms and wonderful changes in their blood cleanliness. The blood sedimentation (toxic wastes and debris) dropped. Cholesterol levels were normalized, even though this controlled fasting plan allowed eggs, butter, milk and cod liver oil. Blood sugar levels "turned to the lower side of normal." One diabetic patient gave up taking insulin. Blood pressure also normalized.

---

[1] *The Natural Way to Health Through Controlled Fasting* (Parker Publishing Company, Inc.), 1968.

The doctors state clearly that "there was a complete curtailment of soft drinks, candy, cake, ice cream or any food made up of white sugar ... Those who felt that the sacrifice of coffee was too great were allowed black coffee—15 minutes before breakfast."

BASIC PLAN

For a period of six months, the arthritics did not eat any foods that contained white sugar; for most of them no coffee. Here are the other diet rules.

1. All daily water intake was consumed solely upon arising, preferably at warm or room temperatures and one hour before breakfast.

2. With meals, the only liquids allowed were room temperature milk or warm soup (not creamed). Throughout the day, these were the only liquids permitted to quench thirst.

3. Cod liver oil, mixed either with 2 tablespoons of fresh, strained orange juice or 2 tablespoons of cool milk was taken at these times:
   (a) One hour before breakfast.
   (b) Thirty minutes after water intake.
   (c) Five hours after the evening meal.
   (d) A short time before retiring for the night.
   Diabetics and those with heart ailments took the oil only twice weekly. All others took the mixture every single day. The cod liver oil mixtures were shaken well in a screw-top glass before taking.

4. Any food supplements or tablets or pills could be taken either with the water upon arising, with milk or soup at mealtime or with milk or soup at any time.

5. No sugar or any sugar-containing food was allowed at any time.

6. No coffee except before breakfast.

This special plan actually washed out the insides of the patients, says Wade, and helped bring about relief and possible cure. In addition to arthritic relief and cure, other benefits were recorded: noticeable skin improvement, better hair and scalp health, cerumen (ear wax) correction, diminishing of inflammatory ear conditions, favorable blood cleansing and urine changes.

The doctors later stated: "We felt these (rapid) improvements were due primarily to the cod liver oil and unusual arrangements for liquid drinking intake. While it is true that these favorable objective and laboratory findings would eventually appear with a favorable diet (alone), the relativity of time to obtain these more or less same results would differ. We obtain our results in three to six months' time. A wholesome diet alone would perhaps take six to 36 months to produce 50 to 75 percent of our results at best."

Each of the major substances in Dr. Campbell's diet is—in itself—a formidable weapon against arthritis. Perhaps that is why the program as a whole is so successful. Take B vitamins, for example:

• Mrs. F.L. said: "I never realized just how badly my ankles, wrists and fingers were swollen until my fingers began to have sharp fleeting pains, especially in the joints (I am a typist, violinist and stenographer). My hands are my livelihood. Vitamin B complex drained off pounds of water; my fingers now look actually 'skinny' and much thinner, and the most important thing, my spirits have lifted tremendously."

• Mrs. H.E. said: "Last year, after spraining my wrist several times, I lost the use of it completely. A prescription for the pain did nothing for the wrist, and made me sleepy ... my doctor gave me a new prescription ... I developed stomachaches ... I still had a sore wrist. I am a writer, and I could not type five minutes without developing the most excruciating pain in my sore wrist ... Then I heard about taking vitamin B-6 for stiffness, and started taking about 50 mg daily. I got excellent results (in a few weeks). Last week I put in six straight hours at my typewriter without a twinge!"

• Liver is rich in B vitamins. One man said: "Eight months ago I bought some dessicated liver, never dreaming it would really do wonders for my health ... I am 53 and my health was failing fast. I had arthritis of the spine in an advanced stage ... In three days, I could jump out of bed without dragging myself ... My friends who had not seen me for months could hardly believe I was the same person they once knew. And do you think I tell them what I have discovered? You bet I do! I have started over 50 people taking dessicated liver. This is what it has done for me. No more pain any more, no nausea, nerves calm, no colitis, no phlegm in my throat and my headaches have stopped."

Calcium starvation has a lot to do with arthritis. As one doctor explained it, in emotional or physical stress—if you lack calcium—your body draws it from the bones. To make up for this, it puts some back at the weakest point, the joints. Excess buildup at the joints causes crippling. Adding lots of calcium to the diet, he says, removes the need for thickened joints. The excess is dissolved or reabsorbed. Unless calcium is supplied, joints continue to thicken.

- In one case, a 30-year-old woman, Candice C., fell and broke her thigh. It was barely healed enough for her to walk on crutches when it broke again. Expensive surgery was done, and she was given a plastic hip joint. After many months of pain, calcium began forming over the plastic bone! Then she tried an eating plan involving generous amounts of calcium. In three days, her pain disappeared completely.

- "About four years ago," said Ms. M.A., "I started to develop arthritis. I consulted six doctors ... no help ... At times I could not even turn a water faucet on ... And then one day I heard that bone meal (calcium) was good for 'bone aches.' I got a bottle and started taking six tablets a day ... I know three months do not make a cure, but I no longer have pains. I can now move easily and I am off pain-killing drugs ... My husband suggested we give some bone meal to our dog, and she also has lost her limp."

Finally, there is iodine, contained in seafood and sea water (the kind sold in health food stores is safe to drink). In one case:

- Kenneth D., 92, was senile and completely crippled with arthritis. He had to be lifted out of bed and could not dress or feed himself. On a doctor's advice, he was given 1 teaspoonful of concentrated sea water per day. Suddenly he began to perk up. After being senile and crippled for many years, he began to get up every morning and fix breakfast. He'd had an arthritic hip for 20 years and would yell if anyone touched it, even gently. But now he crossed his legs to put his shoes on, and let the foot hit the floor without a peep.

Dr. Campbell's diet also contains generous amounts of vitamins A, C, E, sulphur, manganese and potassium, each of which has proven valuable in fighting various forms of arthritis, infection, swelling and catarrhal inflammation.

RAPID HEALING FOODS FOR ARTHRITIS

Alfalfa tea may bring blessed relief and freedom from pain. One man said: "I have had arthritis in my back for years. Three months ago I was so bad I could hardly get in and out of my car. Then I learned of a woman who had cured her arthritis by drinking alfalfa tea. I decided to try alfalfa seeds for my problem. I grind up 3 tablespoonfuls every day and mix with yogurt or milk as part of my lunch. I am delighted that my back is in wonderful shape again."

"I have personally experienced a miracle in my life," said Mrs. A.Y. "For nine years I suffered with rheumatoid arthritis— I lived on aspirin, then cortisone, Indocin, Butazolidin, etc., but not one of these helped. My heart problems were innumerable and I had quite a bit of crippling from arthritis. My weight went down to 96 pounds (I'm 5 feet, nine). I was anemic ... and worst of all, I was in constant, severe pain.

"Then a friend recommended alfalfa tea (four or five times a day). I began drinking it every day (and now at least twice a week). My health improved and the pain lessened every day. Today I live a nearly normal life, my blood count is normal and my weight is 140 pounds. I eat lots of fresh fruits and vegetables and avoid sugar, coffee, overly processed and chemical-laden foods and white flour. Every day I thank God that my life has turned around from a bed-ridden cripple to a useful citizen."

Apple cider vinegar has relieved crippling knee pain. Mrs. A.T. said: "My father had a bad knee from kneeling on cement welding for 20 years. A couple of years ago, it started getting so bad he would miss work and have to stay home with a heating pad on it. The knee would swell to twice its normal size. On one occasion, his knee completely gave out crossing a street and he collapsed on the ground. Doctors gave him pain killers but nothing helped. About a year ago, he began drinking one part apple cider vinegar to two parts water every day. After a couple of weeks, the pain subsided, the swelling completely disappeared and didn't return."

Cherries may bring you amazing relief from arthritis. Ludwig W. Blau, M.D., in *Texas Reports on Biology and Medicine* (vol. 8) tells of an astounding cure among arthritis patients who were given cherry juice. Gout sufferers were especially relieved. No attacks of gouty arthritis occurred on a nonrestricted diet in all cases, as a result of eating about one-half pound of fresh or canned cherries per day. One doctor said: "A patient of mine had heard about cherries for gout. He was, in fact, a sufferer of gout himself. He decided to give the cherry therapy a try. After following this patient's progress over the past two months, I can only say the results have been nothing less than spectacular. The patient has ceased taking the prescribed medication for his gout and has an unlimited diet. This alone should make any gout sufferer take notice. It can't do any harm to try it."

"After hearing about them, I began eating red, sour cherries for my gout," said Mrs. M.G. "I had been taking various drugs, but I still had a lot of swelling. By eating cherries daily, I have been able to leave off medications entirely, and the swelling in my ankles is gone. By adding vitamin E to my diet, the terrible leg pains I was plagued with at night have been greatly reduced also. Through the use of vitamins and food supplements, I have been able to stop using all arthritis medications. This is the first time in 20 years that I have been able to leave off drugs for arthritis."

Garlic has been hailed as a cure for arthritis. This may have something to do with its power to relieve infections, catarrhal swellings and inflammation of the lining of the joints or its well-known power to increase the circulation. An Indian scientist states that garlic oil, used as a liniment, has always been used with great success in paralytic and rheumatic afflictions. Garlic contains sulphur, which fights toxic poisons in the body, and kills germs of putrefaction in the intestines, which drugless doctors believe is the basic cause of arthritic and rheumatic pain.

Honey may relieve arthritis. One woman, crippled with arthritis, had reached the point where she felt she just had to live with it. She moved to a boarding house, where honey was served instead of sugar. Within a short time, she found—to her amazement—that her arthritis had disappeared.

Vitamin C, like vitamin A, fights infections, swelling and catarrhal inflammation. It is also a main ingredient in collagen, the tissue cement that builds strong bones. One doctor, himself a victim of low back and hip pain, recommends 500 mg with every meal to patients with all kinds of ligament, back, hip, neck and arm pain. He says that pain disappears in 24 to 48 hours, and says that 93 percent have had dramatic relief and are able to do heavy work, including hiking and tennis. He says that a large number with disc lesions were able to avoid surgery, and that this will eliminate most common back pains, sprains and disc ruptures. He says that exercise is necessary to help the vitamin reach all parts of the spine. Other specialists caution against large doses (7,000 to 8,000 mg) taken all at once, especially on an empty stomach, which can cause abnormal cell growth, but smaller amounts are not harmful.

One woman said her back was so painful she went to two specialists, and was given exercises and muscle relaxers to take. "Well, the pills were like drinking water and the exercises made it worse," she said. "I gave up in tears. Then I heard about vitamin C for bad backs. I began on 2,000 mg of vitamin C. I must admit I was skeptical at first, but my soreness disappeared in two days. Hallelujah! I have yet to feel the first pain or stiff or sore muscle. I couldn't even get out of bed three months ago."

A man with a slipped disc, told by doctors he'd never get any better, might even get worse, suffered for 20 years in excruciating agony. Then he discovered that when he took vitamin C for a cold, his back stopped hurting. "The next time my neck started to tighten up I took a gram of vitamin C in the morning and another gram at night. The muscles loosened up, and the vertebrae creaked and cracked, going back in place, and I had no more pain. For the last five years I have kept myself free of back pain by taking twice my normal amount of vitamin C every time my neck starts to tighten up."

A woman with a painful heel spur was given pills and ointments, and told to wear a soft pad in her shoe—which did not bring any relief. "I was desperate," she said. "When I read press reports about vitamin C and arthritis, I bought some and started taking 4 or 5 grams a day. On the third day, the heel was not painful to lean on anymore."

In nature, bioflavonoids (vitamin P) are closely associated with vitamin C, and are the major difference between synthetic vitamin C, which does not contain them, and organic vitamin C derived from a natural source like rose hips. "I'm a hairdresser," said Mrs. V.L., "and use my arms a lot. I had bursitis in both arms. Several times I had to have cortisone injected into my shoulders, which was very painful, but the bursitis was more painful. When I heard about vitamin P (bioflavonoids) for bursitis, I bought tablets containing 400 mg of C, 400 mg of citric bioflavonoids and 50 mg of rutin. I took three per day. Within two weeks, there was no more pain. That was three years ago. My doctor told me when I had been cured five years he would give the vitamins credit for it. I have shared this with others; they have had the same results."

Mrs. J.P. said: "Recently, my mother-in-law came for a visit. I was shocked to see how she had deteriorated from arthritis in a very short time. I immediately started her on my 'arthritis formula' as I call it. Each morning she received one vitamin A and D combination perle, 400 I.U. of vitamin E, 500 mg of vitamin C, B complex, 500 mg of pantothenic acid and a calcium tablet. Each afternoon she received another 500 mg of pantothenic acid and another calcium tablet. This was repeated at bedtime. Of course, her diet was changed from 'fast food specials' to balanced meals, no sugar and no white flour. Her coffee intake was reduced from five cups a day to two or three at most.

"At the end of two weeks, this woman—who was pushed and carried up the steps, lifted into and out of the bathtub and sat in the rocker all day—was walking up and down steps with little assistance, doing dishes and getting into the tub herself. She plans to continue her 'formula.'"

Mr. S.V. said: "After years of suffering with a bad knee (a doctor said I had calcium in the soft tissue), I read about niacinamide, a food supplement, for arthritis. I rushed out and bought some. After taking *one tablet* my pain absolutely disappeared, and hasn't returned. I take one (100 mg) whenever I feel the pain, and that is hardly more than one per week.

Vitamin E has been used as follows: "I sprained my shoulder and was given aspirin and codeine for the excruciating pain that made it impossible to get more than two or three hours of sleep a night," Mrs. E.L. said. "The medicine was ineffective, and then I remembered reading about vitamin E for nerve and muscle pain. I decided to try it after experiencing the worst night I'd ever had with my shoulder pain. After the first treatment of vitamin E and calcium, I was pain-free. It was amazing, and a wonderful relief, because I have been able to sleep from six to eight hours at night, pain-free!"

For years, another man suffered from torn ligaments in his knee. Even though he had the best doctors, including a famous specialist who prescribed exercises with weights and arch supports, the pain was still there. Then he started taking vitamin E (600 to 800 units daily). Within a week the pain disappeared. A woman with arthritic knee pain says her doctor recommended a rubber stocking, which had no effect at all. The pain was severe and she couldn't sleep at night. Walking with a cane was painfully difficult, almost impossible. Then she began taking vitamin C, vitamin E, bone meal and dolomite. In about two weeks the pain was entirely gone, to her great joy and amazement. Gradually the stiffness disappeared, and in a month she was walking freely.

One man said: "I suffered with enough pain of an arthritic nature in my right lower limb to last 10 lifetimes ... I needed a cane. I couldn't be without it. Words cannot describe that excruciating pain. The owner of a health food store noticed my cane, and suggested vitamin E. It was like a miracle. In three or four days, the pain in my leg lessened. I stopped the aspirin. In a week, I could walk without a cane or limp. The impossible had happened. Can you imagine my relief? I had suffered 14 years. I have not taken one aspirin in five years."

Zinc may also relieve arthritic pain. "At the age of 83," one man said, "I experienced some pain in both knees. I blamed it on the damp weather, and my age. The pain became worse as time went by and there was now a slight swelling. It became torture every morning to bend my knees to put socks on; and sitting for several hours with friends made it so bad I could barely get up and answer the phone, or walk with my friends to the door. They would kid me with 'old age has finally caught up with you.' Then a miracle occurred. I happened to have some zinc tablets around the house, and rather than waste them I started taking them. To my surprise, I noticed a few weeks later that the pain in my knees had become less severe, and the swelling had gone down some. I began to take a zinc tablet with each meal. In two months the pain and swelling were completely gone. We can't go on blaming every ailment that plagues the elderly on old age. Why was I in misery with my knee at the age of 83, but free of the ailment at nearly 85? Today I can keep stride with my younger friends, kick, jump or run without having any discomfort whatever."

CAUSE AND CURE OF BACKACHES

Strictly speaking, not all aches and pains are arthritic and may be due to other factors. This is especially true of backaches. Backaches stem from a variety of causes, the most common being:

1. Spinal lesions: these are partially dislocated vertebrae which have been pushed out of place on account of muscular weakness. They may be caused in some cases by accidents or faulty posture. Backache from spinal lesions may occur at any part of the spine, and will also irritate other organs of the body, causing pressure on certain nerves.

2. Prolapsed uterus: in women, a sagging uterus, pulling upon ligaments which are attached to the spine, can produce lower back pain, of a persistent dragging-down nature. (See Chapter 12.)

3. Lumbago: lower back pain, in men, usually arises from some disorder of the prostate gland (Chapter 13) or an irritation of the urethra or bladder (Chapter 7). In women, it may stem from uterine or bladder disorders.

4. Inflammation of the bladder: in either sex, inflammation of the bladder is a constant source of distress in the lower back, and a chronic inflammation of the bladder will show more pains in the back than in the bladder itself. (See Chapter 7.)

5. Kidney stones: these stones produce a sharp colicky pain in the right or left side, slightly toward the back. (See Chapter 7.)

6. Muscular weakness: backache may be caused simply by general weakness of the back muscles which have not been sufficiently exercised.

If you are suffering from any form of backache, drugless doctors often recommend some form of body-building regime, in order to be permanently cured (see exercises for the prone position, Chapter 12), under the care of a qualified doctor. These muscle strengthening exercises help slipped discs stay in place.

Sagging abdominal organs, which may be causing backache, are helped by exercises done while lying on the back (see Chapter 12). "I have never seen a case of prolapsed (sagging) stomach or uterus which could not be raised to normal position with these exercises," said one drugless osteopathic doctor.

"If backache is caused by pain from the bladder, it will always be necessary to drink large quantities of water between meals, to keep the urine so diluted that it will not be irritating to the bladder," says this doctor. "Any ache in the lower back will be relieved by applications of hot towels, or a therapeutic lamp, if available. Heat may also be applied through the enema, or through treatment by rectal irrigation. A suitable instrument may be purchased in any surgical supply store, which may be attached to the enema bag, and if this is inserted into the rectum and quantities of hot water allowed to run in and out, it will have a very quick effect in relieving bladder, prostatic or uterine inflammation.

"I find that lumbago, sciatica, rheumatism and pain in the shoulders and arms may often be instantly relieved by applying heat over the bladder and over the lower spine upon those nerves/which carry the nerve impulses to the bladder.

"Much pain in the back is mistaken for rheumatism, when it is only a reflex from an irritated bladder or uterus or prostate gland. In the cure of any form of backache it is well to begin with a general constitutional treatment, and the fasting cure is especially advised in all of those forms of backache which occur in the lower spine. After the diet is resumed, foods which are irritating to the bladder must be avoided."

Reported Cases:

• A 35-year-old woman was suffering from severe pains in the lower back, due to chronic cystitis or inflammation of the bladder. She said she urinated quite frequently, and even had to get up several times a night for this—but was not aware of any other urinary problems. "I told her that her backache was being caused by a bladder which was constantly irritated by urine overloaded with poisonous material," says this doctor. She was placed on a fast for 12 days, using only large quantities of water, without any fruit juice. The backache completely disappeared.

- A man, 62, suffered from lumbago (low back pain) due to an enlarged prostate. This was reduced in two weeks with a plain water fast, and a rectal irrigation twice daily, followed by an enema in the knee-chest position. He used six quarts of water each time, allowing it to run in and out against the prostate. This, combined with fasting, reduced the prostate to practically normal size. The lumbago entirely disappeared after a few days and never returned. (See Chapter 13.)

16

Rapid Healing Foods with Youth Restorative X: The Secret That May Actually Make You Young Again!

Here is the amazing story of Anton L.—the man who grew young at 65! It is based on solid fact. After years of persistent investigation into the causes of physical old age, Anton L. discovered Youth Restorative X—the cleansing and rejuvenation secret revealed in this book, that can wipe out the unpleasant symptoms of aging, restore youth and postpone aging—even in seemingly hopeless cases—for many years.

At 60, Anton L. was a tired, old man. Many years of overeating, hearty drinking and long hours of hard work had taken their toll. He was then wrinkled, balding and quite ill, with agonizing rheumatism and stomach ulcers. He was an old man and looked it. Then a remarkable change of health occurred!

After much research, Anton L. discovered the secret of perfect health and complete freedom from disease, which he called Youth Restorative X. One by one, his physical ailments vanished, and he began enjoying robust and youthful health again—health such as he had not enjoyed in 40 years! In a matter of weeks, with Youth Restorative X, Anton actually started growing younger.

EVENTS THAT CAST SHADOWS!

Medicines and patent remedies only made him suffer more, said Anton. He was chained to them, and his aches and pains returned with a vengeance as soon as he stopped taking them. "Prescription drugs not only suppress symptoms, they cause the body to retain its foul poisons. I never was a healthy man until I realized that fact. Health cannot be found in any drugstore prescription, nor can life be materially prolonged by any medicinal drugs." Only by observing Nature's laws is good health possible, he declared.

CLAIMS EYESIGHT RESTORED!

For many years, Anton was plagued with poor vision. Long hours of work, as a bookkeeper, had ruined his eyes, until finally he was nearly blind. "The light failed," as he put it. He recovered partially by resting completely, and then suffered a relapse. He was unable to read, strong light was painful to his eyes and he stumbled about wearing dark glasses.

Yet with this method, at 65, his sight improved so much he was able to see without glasses, do extensive reading and research and his eyes were no longer painful. "This great improvement in my sight," he wrote, "is certainly directly due to this method."

In studying the problem, Anton found that the action of each eye was controlled by six muscles. Reasoning that it should be possible to strengthen them, here is the method he developed. Relaxing in the evening—or whenever possible—he would look far to the right, then far to the left, then close his eyes tightly as possible several times. Then, with his eyes turned to the right, he would look up and down; then left, and up and down. He would roll his eyes in a wide circle to the left, and look up, and in a wide circle to the right, and look up, and then reverse the procedure. During these drills, he would strike both temples gently, one at a time, with the palm of his hand, to stimulate circulation. Afterward, he would rinse his eyes with plain water.

DARKENS AND RESTORES HAIR!

At 60, Anton was quite bald, and what little hair he had was thin and streaked with gray. At 65, his doctor noted: "The hair has become quite luxuriant. No indications of baldness." With this method, Anton claimed:

New healthy hairs will spring up in place of dead ones, often from the same root! Wherever life remains in the follicles, new hairs will sprout, he said! Anton found it was possible to stimulate the gland that produces hair color by certain simple hand movements. As a result, his hair became much darker!

"If life still remains in the roots of the hair a healthy growth will usually result," he said. "This method is easy and inexpensive, and I know from personal experience that it works. Try it, and I have every reason to believe you can darken and restore your hair!"

Baldness is due to a lack of circulation, said Anton. Tight hats, tension, anything that draws blood away from the scalp will usually result in baldness. Failure to remove dead hairs which impede the growth of new ones can produce baldness, he said. Germs and unsanitary conditions are also contributing factors. Remove the cause, said Anton, and wherever life remains in the roots, new hairs will sprout.

The scalp must be kept clean, he stressed. Like any other part of the body, it is filled with little pores which are constantly eliminating waste matter from the body. This oily dirt and animal filth must be removed, he said, or the pores will be clogged. So don't be afraid of water and good soap.

Thousands lose their hair by failing to keep it clean, said Anton. Use good hot water and a mild soap. Rinse and then douse the head with cold water (see Chapter 17, page 275). Alternate several hot and cold rinses, to stimulate circulation, he explained. Do this at least five or six times, or more. If life still remains in the roots, a healthy growth will usually result. It is the best hair invigorator yet invented, he claimed. Men should do this twice a week; women at least twice a month. Dry the hair thoroughly afterwards, and apply a few drops of oil to produce a healthy gloss.

If the scalp is itchy, use carbolic water to get rid of the germs, he said. To 1 pint of water, add enough carbolic acid to produce a slight tingling sensation when the scalp is wet, he says, and rinse quickly and thoroughly with plain water. This is sure to destroy any scalp germs. It is an excellent and harmless tonic, he claimed, which may be discontinued when the scalp stops itching, in a couple of weeks.

When the hair is falling out many people are afraid to brush or wash it. This is a mistake, said Anton. Dead hairs, like any other decaying matter, must be removed—for the same reason that decayed food is not stored with fresh produce. They are unsanitary, and a menace to vigorous hair growth. To do this, massage the scalp with the tips of the fingers, and gently pull the hair on various parts of the scalp. This stimulates scalp muscles, increases circulation and removes dead hairs. Then wash or comb and brush. Let the sun get at your hair, and avoid wearing hats as much as possible, said Anton. Baldness is almost unknown in certain parts of the world where hats are never worn; whereas in places where tight hats or caps are always donned, baldness or thinning hair is quite common. That is a hint from Nature.

Contrary to popular belief, said Anton, dandruff is a healthy sign. It indicates a healthy growth cycle, and the continual generation of new scalp cells, replacing old, worn-out ones. Dandruff practically ceases when baldness sets in. One of the arguments against washing the hair is that it causes dandruff to appear. The fact is, the dandruff was there before the scalp was washed, and the washing merely loosened it. To be sure, large flakes of dandruff are unsightly. Vigorous brushing will remove them. Have the hair trimmed often, keep it clean, expose the scalp to the sun (see Chapter 18) and dandruff will cease to be a problem.

Anton claimed this method would darken as well as restore hair, because it stimulates the glands, especially the thyroid gland—which can be independently stimulated with throat muscle exercises. After three months, his hair became much darker. For throat muscle exercises, see pages 242-243. For general body movements, to stimulate all glands and organs, see pages 247 to 250.

EVEN IN ADVANCED AGE, YOU CAN FOOL THE CALENDAR— CHEAT TIME OF 20-30 YEARS!

You can restore to the skin the smoothness of youth, said Anton. With this secret wrinkles are erased, youthful shape restored. And this much-to-be-desired condition can be accomplished without cost, he said. You will actually look younger under the closest inspection, he emphasized, and your new look will "stay put" and not "wash off"!

Anton claimed it is possible to erase these lines even in advanced age. At 60, his face was covered with wrinkles, and was drawn and haggard. At 65, his face was smooth and young!

According to all reports, at 65, Anton's face was that of a well-preserved man of 40 or less. His neck was smooth, the neck of a very young man. His throat was no longer loose or hanging, but firm. His chin and cheeks were round and full. In his upper eighties, Anton's face was still remarkably smooth and free of wrinkles.

SMOOTH SKIN RESTORED!

Anton carefully studied the secrets of Ninon de L'Enclos, the great French beauty who, at 90, was still so physically alluring that young men fell hopelessly in love with her! Her face was as smooth and free of wrinkles as it had been at twenty! (This is a well-documented fact.) Her form was as symmetrical, elegant and yielding as a young girl's. Louis XIV declared that she was the marvel of his reign. Ninon declared that anyone could get the same results with this secret!

Authentic pictures of Ninon de L'Enclos at ages ranging from 50 to 85 show a clear, smooth face, with youthful rounded contours, a smooth throat and symmetrical neck that are convincing proof of this method.

Ninon de L'Enclos taught her intimate friends the secret. One of them, Saint Evremond, at the age of 89, was still so handsome that young girls swooned over him! Anton's method for removing wrinkles, filling up hollow cheeks, rounding the chin and smoothing the throat and neck is based on her secret, revealed in an old French pamphlet published in 1710. The author, Jeanne Sauval, was her personal attendant for almost half a century. It is the only successful method for removing wrinkles, said Anton (aside from plastic surgery)!

Specifically, Anton claimed—

* **Eye Lines Disappear!** Lines around the eyes can be erased! This method will strengthen the large circular muscle which surrounds the eye, and when developed will prevent sagginess there. It will also make any hollows in the cheeks fill up and disappear!

* **Chin Firm and Round!** If your chin was ever full and round in youth, that condition will be regained. In Anton's before-and-after pictures, you can see the smooth appearance of youth at age 65, whereas in a picture taken five years earlier, the chin was square and haggard. This improvement takes place rapidly, he says!

* **A Youthful Jaw Line!** If the muscles of the jaw have shrunken, as they usually do in advanced years, the skin will hang loose over them, giving the appearance of age. This method, said Anton, will speedily tone up and increase the size of these muscles, thus giving a rounded and more youthful appearance to the lines of the jaw!

* **Flabby Jowls Vanish!** As years creep on the cheeks sink in and hollows appear where once they were full and plump. This is due to the shrinking of the supporting muscles, and this change produces the hanging or loose jowls and lines of age. With this method, the cheeks fill in, become full and firm, lines disappear, the face becomes smooth. As a means of speedily filling up the cheeks, rounding out the chin, the jaws, no other method will at all compare to it, said Anton. Satisfactory results can be obtained in a very short time, and with very little effort. Results are rapid and astonishing!

* **Mouth Lines Disappear!** The mouth is encircled by a wide muscular band, which grows weaker as we advance in years, causing the mouth to sag and droop at the corners, with deep lines developing. In Anton's full face photos, his mouth does not droop at all, but is as firm as it was when he was 30 years

younger. This method, he says, will speedily firm up the skin around the mouth. Any droop or sagginess will disappear!

● **Crow's Feet Disappear!** With age, the supporting muscles of the temples usually sink and the sunken temples of age appear. This method, says Anton, will produce youthfully smooth temples, and will also remove crow's feet, he promises.

● **How to Erase Wrinkles!** As we advance in years, certain lines appear on the face and neck. First to appear are the wrinkles extending from the nostrils to the corners of the mouth, and beyond. Later, others form at the corners of the mouth, extending down in a curve. Lines on the forehead appear, "crow's feet" spread fanwise from the corners of the eyes. The skin below the eyes becomes loose and creased. Tiny lines appear all over the face and neck, deepen and criss-cross in a tangled web. Here is the only sure method of erasing these lines, says Anton.

● **Sagging Throat Firms Up!** In youth, the throat is graceful and smooth because of a large muscle extending from the voice box to the chin, which is strong and firm at that time. As years creep on, if that muscle is not exercised, it shrinks, and the skin (without support) becomes seamed and wrinkled, and later falls into loose hanging folds. This method brings back the smoothness of youth to the throat!

Anton proved—in his own case—that wrinkles can be removed from the face and neck, even in advanced age. "The deep lines which once criss-crossed my face and neck have entirely disappeared, and my appearance at this point (age 65) is that of a young man half my age," he wrote.

THE REJUVENATION OF THE FACE, THROAT AND NECK!

When muscles are exercised, they become firm and round again. It's as simple as that, said Anton. This applies as much to the face, as any other part of the body. If neglected, these facial muscles will become flabby. If exercised, the hollow places in the neck and cheeks can be filled up, the muscles which surround the eyes can regain the smoothness of youth, to a very considerable extent. The skin can be polished and the wrinkles smoothed out, with the palms of the hands and the tips of the fingers.

The points which will probably first need massaging will be the corners of the eyes and mouth. To prevent chafing, apply some oil to the areas you are rubbing, "skin food" if you please. Any smooth face cream will be just as effective. To avoid soreness, proceed gently and gradually. Stick to it and you will succeed, said Anton.

ROUNDING THE CHIN

Set your teeth firmly, and bunch up your chin muscles. To do this, it helps to stretch or widen the lower lip, exposing the lower front teeth. With the palm of your hand, gently massage the chin. If your chin was ever full and round in youth, the condition will speedily return.

SMOOTHING THE JAW

The jaw muscles readily respond to gentle, rejuvenating massage, said Anton. This should be practiced along the edge of the jaw bone, using the heel of the hand. This treatment will speedily tone up and increase the size of these muscles, thus giving a rounded and more youthful appearance to the lines of the face, he said.

REGAINING
YOUTHFUL CHEEKS

First, contract or bunch up the cheek muscles on one side. Then massage gently with the palm of the hand on this side, upward and well towards the corners of the eyes. Ten or 15 minutes will be sufficient to commence with. Repeat on the other side—or do both simultaneously. This will also prevent bagginess around the eyes, and cause hollows in the cheeks to disappear, said Anton. Drinking plenty of milk will cause an increase of soft, cushiony fatty tissues, and the surface of the skin will be smoother.

REGAINING A YOUTHFUL THROAT

The throat can be smoothed by gently massaging it with the fingers and hands. The throat muscles must be exercised. They are voluntary, and can be exercised at will. Upon them the contour of the face depends. A large muscle extends from the voice box to the lower chin. If not exercised, the throat eventually falls into loose hanging folds. By exercising, this can be reversed, a youthful throat restored, in many cases. Anton did this when he was 60. In a matter of months, the loose folds disappeared. After middle age, even after the half-century mark has been passed, wrinkles will disappear, and much of the smoothness of youth will return, said Anton.

Lay upon your back, a pillow under your shoulders, and let your head fall back as far as possible. Then lift and lower your head. Begin slowly. Start with about five movements. Day by day, increase it. Soon you can attain 100 or more with ease—that is, throwing the head backward as far as possible and then bringing it forward. Rapid results are achieved this way, said Anton. You will round out the neck, and disfiguring bags will disappear. If the throat is too fat and full, this exercise will speedily reduce it.[1]

SMOOTHING OUT THE NECK

If the neck muscles are poorly developed, lines will eventually develop, criss-crossing around the back. Gently massaging the neck with the palms of the hands will, to a considerable extent, erase those wrinkles, said Anton. Lying on your back, alternately raise and lower your head five or 10 times. Clasp the hands firmly behind the head, raise the head clear of the pillow and press backward, exerting a strong forward, or resistance pressure with the arms. Start with five movements and gradually increase to 25. Lying on your side, turn the chin as far as possible towards the upper shoulder. Start with five movements on each side and gradually increase to 10 or 20. These movements will improve the contour of the throat, and erase neck lines, said Anton.

REGAINING A YOUTHFUL MOUTH

The mouth is encircled by a wide muscular band. As we advance in years, if that muscle is not exercised, it will atrophy

---

[1]There is another advantage. Raising the head forward contracts the abdominal muscles, which relax when the head is dropped again. This has a very beneficial effect on the digestive organs.

and, becoming weaker, the mouth will sag and droop at the corners—deep lines will then extend from those points downward, the result being the slack mouth of age. To prevent this, Anton inserted his little fingers at the corners of his mouth, alternately pulling and relaxing. The result was that his mouth became as smooth as it was when he was 35.

ERASING SUNKEN TEMPLES
AND CROW'S FEET

With age the supporting muscles of the temples usually sink and "the sunken temples of age" appear. They should be developed and filled up by gentle massage, which will remedy the trouble, said Anton. Massaging well toward the eyes is advisable, he said. It will produce the smooth temples of youth and will also remove crow's feet.

REJUVENATING THE SKIN

Anton recommended massage of the face and neck, to remove wrinkles. This works mainly by making the facial muscles smooth and round again. This can be done with the bare hands. However, Anton preferred to use goat-hair friction mittens or a goat-hair friction belt. Afterward, he recommended that the face and neck be washed with tepid water softened with borax. He also recommended the use of egg white as a very effective and very cheap method of removing wrinkles, while waiting for the underlying muscles to firm up. This works as an astringent for toning up or shrinking the loose skin of age. It should be done after massaging the face and neck. To understand how it works, you may remember "grandmother's method" of "bringing a boil to a head." She simply pasted the skin of an egg evenly all over the boil. In about 15 minutes, the egg skin began to shrivel, drawing the boil to a head. It also tones up the skin. Try it on the skin of your hand.

Anton's method is based on the same principle, only the liquid white is used as skin food. When it dries, it too becomes a kind of skin. In the drying process it shrinks evenly all over. It is a powerful wrinkle remover. Apply this liquid white all over your face wherever wrinkles appear, said Anton, using a shaving brush for convenience. Then let it dry and remain for five minutes. It is such a strong astringent that it should remain on the skin only a short time, as it may otherwise cause the skin to shrivel. Then rinse it off with pure, warm water. It will readily dissolve and you will be surprised at the smoothness of your skin. If any irritation is felt, apply a few drops of cream, and wipe clean.

HOW YOUTH RESTORATIVE X CAN MAKE YOU YOUNGER!

Anton claimed his secret was a major breakthrough in reversing hardening of the arteries, which he said is the principal cause of "old age." As we advance in years, he said, there is a clogging up of the arteries by chalky deposits. These deposits are somewhat similar to the crust that develops in a water pipe or drain after prolonged use. When this happens, the pipe soon becomes clogged up and useless, but when cleaned it again resumes its former efficiency.

In the same way, when the arteries carrying blood to the organs become clogged, the blood supply diminishes. Organs deteriorate. That is old age. The blood supply to the brain becomes less and less, for example, and the vigorous brain of youth gives way to loss of memory, confusion and senility. But if the human body can be kept free of worn-out tissues, dead cells or other clogging matter, it will again resume the conditions of youth.

If the arteries are open and free of sludge, the heart will pump blood through them easily, and all vital organs will regain their vigor, and the body will appear youthful even at an advanced age. These poisons can be forced out by simple body movements, actually "pumped" out, said Anton. These simple movements, done in bed, will expel that rust or clogging debris, and then you will feel "limbered up," "good as new" again.

YOUTH RESTORATIVE X REVEALED

Youth Restorative X is any method that forces out from the body any waste matter which has accumulated in the venous and glandular system, so it can be carried off by ordinary bodily excretions. In this case, it is a series of alternate contractions and relaxation of certain muscles, done easily while lying in bed.

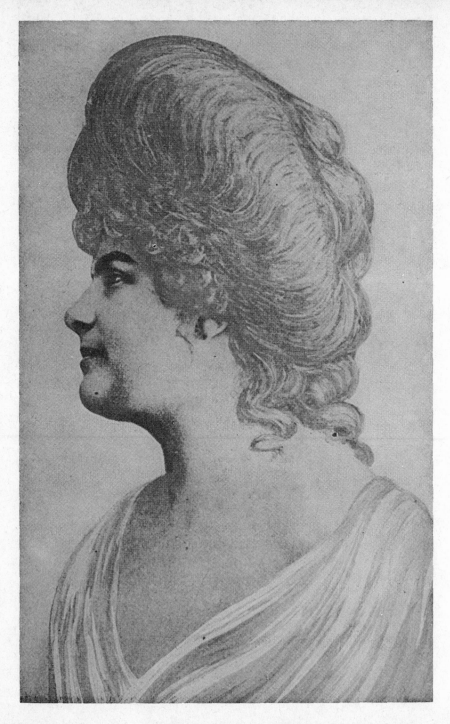

Ninon de L'Enclos at 70.

Here is a clear account of how, at age 60, Anton L. claimed, "I have thrown off the conditions of age, and have become, physically, a young man again." Called Youth Restorative X, it can be accomplished without the use of medicines of any kind, and has the advantage of being without cost.

This method, said Anton, if faithfully followed, will result in improved circulation, healthy glandular activity and will materially prolong your life.

CLAIMS RHEUMATISM DISAPPEARED!

At 65, Anton claimed, "I feel as free and flexible as I did at 25. There is no longer any trace of pain, and the rheumatism I suffered for so long is gone. There is new bounce in my legs, new spring in my step. All this happened in a matter of weeks, and I have been pain-free for five years!"

The basic cause of rheumatism is uric acid in the muscles and joints, which accumulates faster than the body can eliminate it. This uric acid is the result of wrong eating habits, and muscular inactivity. Bread, cake, greasy fried foods, sugars and starch are the principal causes. Yet Anton loved these things and could not bear to give them up. He always drank beer or wine with his meals and ate anything he wanted.

At 60, however, crippled with arthritic pain in his arms and legs, he sought a cure and found it in these simple body movements, which permitted him to "eat his cake and have it." These movements force the uric acid these rich foods produce to move on and be eliminated by the natural body excretions. Uric acid crystals in muscles and joints are dissolved and "pumped" or flushed out.

- Lying upon your back, strike your elbow across your chest. This motion will bring into action the muscles covering the shoulder blades, and will agitate or pump out any acid accumulations in case of rheumatism in the shoulders, said Anton. Do this five times with each arm, he suggested.
- Lying on your back, a small 2-pound weight in each hand, punch at the ceiling (this can be done without the weights, too). Commence with 10 strokes, and increase as your strength improves to 50 or more. It is a safe and effective exercise, said Anton.

- Lying on your back, extend your arms outward, full-length, and turn your wrists back and forth, so that each shoulder will revolve in its socket. If you have rheumatism in your shoulders, where uric acid frequently accumulates, this movement will relieve it, said Anton. Start with five movements and gradually increase to 25, he suggested.

- Lying on your back, grasp the left elbow with the right hand, and the right elbow with the left hand, and pull, forcing your shoulder blades apart. Now shrug your shoulders. Start with five movements, increasing daily, until you have reached 25 with ease, without any soreness.

- Lying on your back, each hand grasping the opposite elbow, raise your right shoulder upward and forward as far as possible. Repeat with your left shoulder. Commence with five movements on each side. Gradually increase to 25, when soreness has disappeared.

These simple body movements, done in bed, effortlessly and without strain, pump out accumulated uric acid in muscles and joints. With the uric acid gone, pain will vanish, and this may even effect a cure not possible with drugs, said Anton.

THE SECRET OF NEW YOUTH!

This series of body movements—plus a few more to be described shortly—is the whole basis of Anton's secret of rejuvenation. These movements are all perfectly safe, he said, and will not only relieve arthritic or rheumatic aches and pains, but will clean out veins and arteries and flush the system of poisons by a kind of "pumping" process.

That is the secret of getting young again—physically—says Anton. If you neglect to flush out clogging ashes in your system, the waste by-product of living, your body will surely stiffen and become rusty, just like any other piece of machinery, he says, and you will show all the common signs of aging.

These simple movements are all done while lying in bed. And as all the movements are done slowly, the bed-clothes need not even be ruffled, neither will the pulse be accelerated. This method of lazy stretching can help you—without strain—expel that rust or clogging debris, and then you will feel limbered up.

And you will live much longer than if your body was in a rusty, clogged-up state, said Anton.

- Lying on your back, arms folded across your chest, raise your head and shoulders and bend to one side. Then back and down and relax. Do this twice on each side, gradually increasing to five times, as you feel up to it.

- Lying on your side, bend your hip and knee forward. Do this three times on each side, increasing gradually to 25. This exercise is valuable in cases of constipation. It reduces a "pot belly" and greatly reduces the possibility of rupture (from any sudden strain) when the lower abdominal muscles are weak.

- Lying on your side, raise your head and both feet at the same time. This will tense muscles running from the arms to the hips. It will also strengthen the stomach. Start with three movements, on each side. Gradually increase to five or six, if you can, in a few days.

- With your arms folded, first on your back—then on each side—stretch until your whole body becomes rigid. Hold this position for two or three seconds. Relax for a few seconds; then repeat. Do this three or four times. Increase slowly, over a period of several days, until you have reached 10.

- Lying on your side, hold your left knee with your left hand, and pull. Hold it a few seconds, then relax. Reverse position. Begin with 10 movements on each side, gradually increasing to 25. This stretches your shoulder muscles across and downward, and strengthens the back.

- Lying on your side, hold one knee with both hands and pull hard for a few seconds, then relax. Begin with 10 movements on each side. This strengthens the back, shoulders and hips.

EASY-DOES-IT!

Go slow with these exercises. Easy-does-it is the rule. They are meant to be done slowly. It is a simple method for those in advanced years whose only aim is health. And such people should confine themselves to the few simple movements Anton L. advises. Don't try to learn and practice them all at once. Go slow and practice each one a few times before you take up the next, on successive days.

- Lying on your side, hold the fist of one hand in the palm of the other and push them together. Turn over and repeat. Do this five times on each side, gradually increasing to 10 or 15.
- Lying on your side, clasp your hands and pull them apart, turning the wrists slightly back and forth. Begin with 10 movements, on each side, and increase gradually, every day, until you feel tired.
- Lying on your back, extend your arms downward, clenching your fists, and turn the arms inward five times, then outward five times. Gradually increase to 10 times.
- Lying on your side, hold your upper arm and pull in opposite directions. Do this five times on each side.
- Lying on your side, slowly "walk," swinging your upper leg and upper arm as far backward and forward as possible. Do this as many times as you wish, but avoid fatigue.

Do not neglect the following methods (even if you feel they do not pertain to you). Rather, add them to your rejuvenation program. Anton practiced them all.

THE SECRET OF GOOD DIGESTION!

Anton had much to say about indigestion, as he suffered from a long list of ailments, ranging from ulcers to a sluggish liver and constipation. Yet all these ailments disappeared, for good, in a matter of weeks, when he adopted the following system. First, said Anton, take more time at meals. Don't gulp your food. Chew it thoroughly. This one change alone will quickly improve your digestion, he said. If you smoke after meals, don't do it, he cautioned. Wait until your food is thoroughly digested, if you must smoke. Anton loved a good cigar, but waited several hours after eating, to give his system a chance to settle down. Until he discovered this secret, he suffered continual heartburn. Afterwards, the heartburn disappeared for good.

His next suggestion was that if you suffer indigestion, go without solid foods at breakfast. Digestion is very slow when you are sleeping, and if you have eaten a heavy supper, your body may be still working hard to digest it. It cannot accept more food at this time. If you are accustomed to drinking coffee, or weak tea, at breakfast, and they agree with you, continue to do so, but not even a crust of bread. You'll see a great improvement in a short time, he said.

Copious water drinking—especially a glass about 15 minutes before breakfast—is a good remedy for constipation, said Anton. The next step is to strengthen the muscles of the stomach.

Lying on your back, bend your head well forward. This will tense the abdominal muscles. Let your head fall back to the normal position, and these muscles will relax. As you alternately raise and lower your head, gently thump your fists against your abdomen, several times in rapid succession. After several weeks, as these muscles grow stronger, hit harder. This will produce healthy circulation and strengthen the digestive organs. Also, massage the abdomen, as you would after a full meal. These two methods are harmless, inexpensive and far more effective than any drugs, said Anton.

Internal cleansing was an important part of Anton's system. Animals eat grass when they are constipated, but no other animal on earth eats the vast amount of starchy, processed, gluey foods (breads and pastry) that humans do, nor do they eat for recreation. The enema is the only logical solution, said Anton. Otherwise, this sludge accumulates faster than it can be eliminated, and leaves a hardened residue, which may be irritating, cancer-causing and, at the very least, cause little pockets to form (diverticulitis) or an enlarged intestine. Anton felt that an ordinary enema does not do much good. It takes at least 4 quarts of water to thoroughly wash the colon, he said. In this manner, it can be cleansed without the slightest effort, in about 15 minutes. Do this once or twice a week, to prevent your insides from becoming clogged with fecal matter, the breeding ground of many diseases.

REMEDY FOR A SLUGGISH LIVER!

For 30 years, Anton complained of chronic indigestion, a belching, bitter taste, pains on the right side, gas, headache, dizziness, nausea, foul breath, constipation, chills, perspiration, drowsiness after meals and heart palpitations, all common symptoms of liver and gall bladder problems.

With this method, said Anton, all symptoms of a sluggish liver disappeared. Think of the liver, simply, as a filter through which blood must pass to be freed of its impurities—and as the organ that manufactures bile for breaking up fat. To be healthy, the liver must be exercised, said Anton. This happens naturally, when you are slender and active. For heavy or sedentary people, it should be agitated or massaged by hand. This is best done in the morning, in bed, when the stomach is empty. It is safe and harmless, said Anton.

- Lying on your back, place your fingers below your ribs, on the right side, just above the hip bone, and gently press upward, under the rib. Relax the pressure, and repeat. Use the fingers of both hands, simultaneously. Do this gently about 10 or 20 times, to begin with, increasing as desired.

- Lying on your right side, bend your knees, and press the knuckle of your left thumb well under the ribs on the right side, and massage or agitate, as in the preceding example.

- Lying on your left side bang gently, but rapidly, with your right hand over the liver. Start with 20 light blows, increasing this number as your condition improves.

RELIEVING VARICOSE VEINS!

In varicose veins, a steady upright position produces stagnation of blood in the legs, and pressure on veins, which enlarge. This cannot be cured by lotions or medicines. Surgery is expensive and painful. Temporary relief can be obtained with an elastic stocking, but the trouble returns. The first sign of trouble is a dull, aching pain. The vein becomes much larger, knotted and distended, and sometimes bursts.

- **Anton said this method is a sure cure in any ordinary case. At 40, he developed a painful, bulging varicose vein which annoyed him for the next 20 years. It was always annoying, and threatened to ulcerate or form a clot. For years, he wore an elastic stocking.**

- **Relief is obtained by this method, said Anton. It will relieve the congestion, and restore the distorted venous valves to their proper position, when the trouble will** disappear. It is a simple, easy and very effective remedy for this very annoying condition, he said.

● At 65, Anton's legs were so healthy, he could do a 100-yard dash in nine seconds. He ran a mile in 7:50 without any distress, which he could not do at age 40! "I do not approve of such strenuous effort after middle age," he said, "but was willing to give the demonstration to show the effects of this method." His heart beat returned so quickly to normal that a very able doctor declared he was as fit as a healthy young man half his age.

To relieve the congestion, and accelerate the flow of blood, Anton recommended massage. **Do not do this if you have a clot in your leg, or phlebitis. As with all methods described in this book, check with your doctor first, and get his approval.** In the morning, said Anton, while still in bed and relaxed, lay on your side and gently massage up and down, with the palm of your hand, over the vein. Do this about 20 times, increasing over a period of days or weeks to 100, said Anton.

HOW TO CLEAR THE LUNGS!

Anton said: "My mother died of consumption at 38. I inherited her weak lungs, and throughout my sickly, feeble childhood, I suffered from asthma and bronchitis. Everyone said I would surely go as my mother did. Yet today at 65, I am hale and hearty. I have come back from a gasping, wheezing invalid, plagued with respiratory ailments to one who is absolutely free from coughs, colds or any lung weakness. I strongly urge that you use this method for lung health."

First, see that your home is well-ventilated. Try to walk outside, at least once a day, in the fresh air, inhaling deeply, slowly and as much as possible without any feeling of dizziness. Exhale slowly, and practice this as much as possible in the sunlight (see Chapter 18). As you lie in bed in the morning, practice this same deep breathing exercise.

"With Youth Restorative X, you need not fear pulmonary diseases," said Anton. "By this lung strengthening method, I have increased my chest expansion and doubled my lung capacity. After using this secret myself, I can confidently state that only good will result."

HOW TO CURE A COLD!

Anton L. claimed he had a sure cure for colds that relieved them quickly—almost overnight! As a young man with weak lungs and a tendency to respiratory ailments, he dreaded catching a cold. It always meant a long period of illness, for he recovered very slowly from such attacks. On one occasion, when he caught an "awful cold," he discovered how to get rid of it.

A doctor who did not believe in medicines advised him to use this simple remedy: "Don't eat. Drink all the water you can, but do not take any food. Continue until your temperature returns to normal, in about 48 hours. Go to bed and stay there. If anyone tells you you must eat, don't do it. Do as I tell you."

"I took his advice," said Anton. "The results were exactly as he said. In two days, I was entirely recovered, without any trace of a bad cold. It was amazing, because I fully expected a two-week siege, and here I was, completely well. And this is how I have cured my bad colds ever since for the past 40 years. The proven fact is, this method does cure colds quickly, without expensive drugs. It is one of the reasons why my lungs are so healthy today, at 65." With this quick and easy cure for "bad colds," the clogging rubbish is burned up or eliminated from the body and glandular structures. It also clears up serious sinus problems quickly. And in the early stages of pneumonia, a cure is almost certain, said Anton.

A WORD OF ADVICE

Anton L. concluded by saying: "I have been an old man, and now at 65 I am young again, and look it. Really, I am now in better shape than I was at 35. My trouble now is that nobody believes I'm nearing 70. The physical ailments that plagued me have long since gone. I feel absolutely certain that what I have done you can do. You will probably succeed far more rapidly than I have done. I had to pioneer my own way. And now at 65 I present the appearance of a man little more than half my age. What I accomplished is possible to almost anyone. Follow my example, and success will be yours."

17

Rapid Healing Foods for Relief of Grievous Ailments!

Nearly a century ago, Father Sebastian Kneipp, a humble priest turned healer, grew famous in the little town of Worishoffen, Bavaria, for his knowledge of Rapid Healing Foods, still available everywhere today, without prescription. Of all the foods favored by this priest, one he valued above all others. He regarded this amazing, common natural liquid as Nature's All-Purpose Miracle Remedy for the relief of grievous ailments—water! With the use of this one simple food, a wide range of ailments were quickly cured!

The town grew from a village of 500 to 15,000—with elaborate buildings erected to accommodate the patients of Father Kneipp. From all over the world, thousands came on pilgrimages—the aged, the paralyzed, the sick and those afflicted with all manner of illness—to seek his famous treatments. Afterwards, they were relieved of their ills, rejuvenated and healed! With Rapid Healing Foods thousands of seemingly hopeless cases were cured. Miracles of healing were reported!

"Without my wishing it and without advertisement," said Father Kneipp, "the sick people came in such numbers that we knew not what to do with them. At first I used my own washhouses in which to apply my remedies but as these no longer sufficed, two bath-houses were built above the Village, one for men and one for women. The time soon came when these two buildings were insufficient."

The most remarkable thing was the effect of water upon people of all ages, many of whom arrived half lame, half blind, half deaf, said Father Kneipp, while others were diseased from head to foot.

"Those who do not consider water and herbs sufficient for the healing of the sick cannot rightly know their power," said Father Kneipp. "A proof that water and herbs suffice is given by the thousands of invalids who have found and still find here relief or cure for those illnesses which had been declared past help."

NATURE'S ALL-PURPOSE MIRACLE REMEDY!

Father Kneipp insisted that blood obstructions are the main cause of disease. "When these obstructions occur in various parts of the body, the blood remains as it were cooped up, neither able to advance nor to retire properly," he said. The principle behind the use of water for disease symptoms is simple: water temperature can affect circulation—increase or reduce it at will. This is especially important when tissues and organs are inflamed, or congested.

CIRCULATION INCREASED—SWELLING RELIEVED!

This liquid can rapidly increase circulation in the legs or any other part of the body ... relieve swelling ... clean out clogged veins and arteries. Many years ago it was a miracle youth restorative for elderly people with hardening of the arteries or other circulatory ailments.

When cold water strikes the foot, for example, the blood in that extremity tends to be hurried up the leg by the contracting action of the small blood vessels stimulated by the cold. Immediately, a fresh new supply of blood pours in to take the place of the blood which had been flowing sluggishly. New supplies of life-giving oxygen and cell food are supplied to the tissues of the foot by means of this rapid exchange; cells are cleansed, stimulated and revitalized. Try it some time when your ankles are swollen from tiredness at the end of a day.

What applies to the foot is equally true of any other part of the body. No one needs to be told that a quick dash of cold water to the face brings a healthy glow and is a positive tonic. The same reaction occurs in the legs, chest, back or arms—anywhere that cold water is used to bring a new rush of good blood.

CLEANS OUT CLOGGED VEINS AND ARTERIES!

With the simplest use of running water, you can drive blood more rapidly through sluggish arteries and veins in congested tissues. Yet perhaps not one person in a hundred knows how to use his own bathtub or shower for definite health purposes. To the majority, water is only a cleansing agent or something to drink.

A MIRACLE YOUTH RESTORATIVE!

At Father Kneipp's health spa, every patient had to appear for his water treatment in the morning. For some who were elderly or afflicted with hardened arteries or some other circulatory disturbance, the nozzle of the hose was turned to a spray which fell upon them like soft rain. The temperature of the water was about that of a midsummer shower and the gentle patter on their pallid skins really helped to circulate the blood. Because of the dilation and contraction of the skin arteries, circulation throughout the entire body was greatly stimulated without causing any overload on the heart.

HARDENED ARTERIES REALLY SOFTENED!

And so, perhaps, after a few weeks of gentle water application, hardened arteries were really softened. At least they were much more flexible. Old men whose yellowed skin at first had no glow during a water treatment would begin, within a short time to feel like youngsters. Their skin would be pink as a baby's after their spray bath.

LIVER AILMENT CURED!

The type of spray varied with the individual. A few years ago, a medical doctor who still used water treatments, recalled the case of Mr. J., in his early fifties, who had an early case of hardening of the liver. With this amazing liquid and other Rapid Healing Foods, all symptoms gradually cleared up. He was a prodigious drinker, and a heavy eater, too. His liver was perhaps 25 percent larger than normal, and already showed nodular changes which betokened a typical hobnail liver in the not-too-distant future.

This man was given "blitz" baths by an attendant. This meant turning the nozzle of the hose until there was one straight forceful stream of water, perhaps three-eighths of an inch in diameter. The force of the water was turned on full blast and the temperature, starting out warm, was gradually increased in about three minutes to cold. Only the man's back and legs were "blitzed."

WHISKY NOSE A SYMPTOM OF EARLY HARDENING OF THE LIVER (AND SWELLING OF THE LEGS)

The peculiar thing was that while the gentleman had some of the most uncomfortable symptoms of liver trouble and swelling of the legs, he was mainly concerned over his red nose. It was a typical "whisky" nose, as people call it. He was told that his red nose was a symptom of early hardening of the liver and that it would be red as long as the liver was congested and pathological. Mr. J. did not like the idea of taking "blitz" baths at all.

MIRACLE CLEANSING FOODS USED!

Mr. J. had already been put on a rigid diet, consisting chiefly of fruits and salad vegetables. He had been starved for minerals and vitamins despite his liberal eating, and had a severe case of constipation. All these symptoms gradually cleared up with rapid healing, rapid cleansing foods.

HOW THE WATER CURE HEALED
HIS LIVER!

After a short time, Mr. J. really began to like the blitz baths. Ten to 12 minutes weren't enough. He was willing to stay half an hour and he couldn't see why a little more wouldn't help him. He "went on the wagon," really watched his diet and made splendid progress.

In a few weeks, he was pronounced cured. His nose was no longer red, his "whisky" nose was a thing of the past. Anatomically and functionally, his liver was perfect—even though most doctors agree that once the liver has begun to harden, nothing can be done about it.

POWER TO CONTROL YOUR CIRCULATION!

Years before modern drugs, drugless doctors knew that a stream of water on a man's leg would bring blood there, on a certain part of his back would take blood out of his liver, another at the back of his neck would do something else. With substantial control of the circulation of the blood, with the power to bring blood to whatever part of the body desired, or to take it away, many seemingly hopeless cases were cured.

NO SPECIAL EQUIPMENT NEEDED!

Ordinary garden hoses and the plainest of tubs produce results equal to those effected by the fanciest equipment. Dozens of the simple baths described in this chapter are powerful therapeutic agents. Their cost is negligible. The reason they are not commonly used is that most people never heard of them. Yet they work as well today as they did nearly a century ago, when thousands were helped!

AMAZING RELIEF FOR
HIGH BLOOD PRESSURE!

Hot baths, when properly taken, are very helpful to individuals suffering from high blood pressure. This does not imply that such water treatments are in any way a cure for high blood pressure, which is always a symptom of trouble and not a disease in itself. This amazing liquid, in the form of hot baths, draws blood to the skin, thus relieving blood pressure and tension in the large arteries and internal blood vessels. It can reduce blood pressure as much as 15 points in one sitting.

Relief is long-lasting: the reduction stays in effect from two to six hours, said one medical doctor. In conjunction with rest, baths provide the quickest, and most effective way to lower blood pressure without harm to the body, he said.

NEW BLOOD FOR OLD—
A REMEDY FOR ANEMIA!

Throughout the history of natural medicine, even as far back as Hippocrates, a certain water treatment called the knee bath was known as a remedy for anemia. The earliest practitioners filled small wooden tubs with hot water, and added a few heated rocks to keep the liquid from cooling too rapidly. The patient stepped into the water and sat down on a stool right next to the tub. As the legs were thus heated up to the knee, the skin became red. The ancients figured that the flush was caused by a creation of more blood—and termed the bath an anemia remedy.

We know today that they were right in practice and not far wrong in theory. Three physicians working at the University of Chicago made experiments in 1936 which proved that this remedy produces an increase in new blood cells. (The heat stimulates the long bone marrow.) This can help anemia, we are told.

The vindication of this age-old custom by scientific proof means that the knee bath without the hot rocks and in a modern bathtub is still an excellent and costless method of stimulating the formation of needed blood cells. It is especially valuable for those with simple anemia, or those who have experienced temporary loss of blood.

AMAZING RELIEF FOR ARTHRITIS,
RHEUMATISM, GOUT, SWOLLEN FEET!

Water treatment, in the form of the hot submersion bath, is of tremendous importance to the comfort of an arthritis victim, and to his ability to use crippled fingers and limbs once more. Its principle is the same as that of the underwater exercise given to victims of paralysis. Lessened external pressure under water enables the individual to move joints much more easily. The heat of the submersion bath produces a slight rise in temperature, hence the name "fever" bath. Years ago, most doctors considered fever a deadly enemy, to be reduced by any means and at any cost. Now we know what Hippocrates believed 2,000 years ago is true: that fever is one of Nature's ways of fighting infection, of stimulating blood supply and promoting healing. Even cavemen knew this liquid could relieve arthritic pain.

The whole idea of hot or sweat baths for relief of arthritic and rheumatic pains is as old as history. Cavemen probably availed themselves of heated water to reduce pain. Certainly, North American Indians learned long ago to use natural hot springs. The remains of Celtic baths, predating the Roman occupation, have been found in Great Britain and Ireland.

The procedure of the submersion bath is simplicity itself. Merely fill a bathtub as full as possible with hot water. Submerge the affected part, and try to move the joints back and forth. Soon, practically no pain is felt under the hot water, and after a few experiences, the joints move much more easily. Such movement aids blood circulation through the painful areas, and is of definite therapeutic value, said one medical doctor. Best results are obtained by using water as hot as can be borne, to take one or two baths a day and rest in bed for a short time afterwards, he said.

This medical doctor also recommended the following:

- FOR HEADACHES: for the common type of throbbing headache, when the head is full of blood, undress, run about 8 inches of very cold water into the bathtub, and squat in it until it covers the hips. Count to 10, then get out. Dry the body and lie down for a few minutes. The congestion will be gone from the aching head; so will the pain.

- ANEMIC HEADACHES: for the so-called anemic type headache, accompanied by facial paleness and a dull, continuous pain chiefly in the back of the head, undress, run 8 inches of very hot water in the bathtub and sit in it slowly. Recline for about 10 or 15 minutes, then get out, dry yourself and lie down. The pain will have been relieved as if by magic.

- MIGRAINE HEADACHES: as an aid in relieving the intense symptomatic pain of migraine, the hot half-bath is a most effective measure. Undress, run about 8 inches of hot water in the bathtub and squat in it for 15 or 20 minutes. When the blood has been drawn out of the head into the legs or hips, the severity of the headache usually decreases. At the first sign of a headache, take only fruit juices the rest of the day and cleanse the bowels, and suffering will be greatly relieved.

- FOR HEMORRHOIDS: sit in enough cold water to cover the hips completely, and knead and rub the abdomen. Dry with a coarse towel, then rub and pat the skin with the hands for a few minutes.

- FOR VARICOSE VEINS: stand in cold water up to the knees or calves, from one to two minutes, then dry skin with a coarse towel and rub vigorously with the hands, or walk about briskly for a few minutes. Repeat as needed.

- FOR HAIR GROWTH: if the hair is short, the head should be washed thoroughly with cold water each time the face is washed, vigorously pinching, kneading and massaging the scalp with the fingertips. If the hair is long, dip fingertips in cold water and rub vigorously into scalp.

- FOR PELVIC CRAMPS OR PROSTATE TROUBLE: sit in 4 to 6 inches of lukewarm water or wet a cloth and draw it up between the legs like a diaper and attach it in front and back to a belt around the waist. Extra cold compresses may be inserted inside the cloth, if needed, in inflammation of the rectum and genito-urinary organs.

- FOR HARDENED ARTERIES IN LEGS: turn cold water on full force from a hose, and direct it first on one foot, then the other. Let the stream play alternately on the upper part of the feet and on the soles. The coldness and force of the water will draw blood to the feet.

- FOR HOT FLASHES: stand in a bathtub containing about 2 inches of cold water, step and splash vigorously for several minutes, then dry and rub the feet, and increase the circulation by walking around for a few minutes.

- FOR SORE THROAT, SINUSITIS, TONSILLITIS, HOARSENESS: dip a soft piece of cloth in cold water, wring it out and wrap it around the throat. This is excellent in cases of sore throat, tonsils and glands.

- EYE COMPRESSES: a cold, wet compress is very effective for relieving congestion and inflammation in the eyes. Dip cloth in cold water and apply over the eyes. Hold in place by a dry covering.

HOT VERSUS COLD

Father Kneipp favored lightning-fast cold water treatments of a few seconds at most, on various parts of the body. By cold, we mean the normal room temperature of tap water, and certainly not ice water. He felt that while warm water is beneficial in certain cases, it is ultimately weakening to the body, causing relaxation and flabbiness of muscles, veins and arteries. Cold water, on the other hand, he repeatedly stressed, is bracing and strengthening.

For cold water applications to work, said Father Kneipp, the body must be as warm as possible: "He who takes the application with perspiration trickling from every pore will derive the greatest benefit ... He who is only half warm will derive little or no benefit from an application of water."

More specifically, he stated:

"In order to get good results the body must, as we have said, be warm before taking the bath and it must be thoroughly warm as quickly as possible after taking it. This is one of the most important points in the water cure. He who is unaccustomed to water must take double care to regain his natural warmth as quickly as possible either by outdoor exercise or walking up and down in a warm room...

"As far as possible the baths should be taken in the morning. If, however, one is obliged to take them in the afternoon, let it be an hour or two after the midday meal or an hour or two before supper. A bath may be taken with advantage at night after the first sleep, when the body is thoroughly warm and somewhat rested, if the person goes back to bed at once...

"How long is a bath to last? I say the shorter the better; the usual time is from one to two seconds; only on very rare occasions from five to six ... remaining too long in the water destroys its efficacy and tortures the body..."

Oddly enough, cold water actually has a warming effect on the body, by causing vigorous circulation on the part treated. In Bavaria, snow baths and various cold water applications were used by peasants, for their warming effect. Cold water, of course, must be used with caution by the very young and those of advanced years, avoiding sudden shocks to the system.

Father Kneipp recalled:

"A lady of high rank came to me this year; she was somewhat old and so emaciated and feeble as to be scarcely able to walk;

she begged that I would at first use tepid water as she had herself commenced by taking warm footbaths. I gave her a gentle thigh douche of quite cold water, the effect of which was quickly to give warmth. After this she never used warm water, because she gained more warmth and strength from cold, thus confirming my statement that cold water is best ... in applying douches to various parts of the body, use care and gentleness..."

Father Kneipp declared that "the means employed to restore a sick man to health must be of a dissolving and eliminating character in order to rid the body of all its morbid and impure elements. Water is exactly adapted to act upon the body in various ways, and the simplest applications are washings or ablutions..."

HEALING BATHS THAT HAVE STOOD THE TEST OF TIME!

At Father Kneipp's health spa, washings—or ablutions— were used for the whole body, the upper part of the body and the lower part of the body. The first consisted of washing every part of the body from head to foot, so that not a spot was left untouched by the water. The second consisted of washing down to the waist, not including the hair (which once wet dries slowly and is apt to give cold). The third took in the lower part of the body, from the thighs down to the feet. A large sponge or a coarse towel was used—Father Kneipp preferred the latter.

"The first thing of importance," said Father Kneipp, "is to get it over as quickly as possible. The washing of the whole body should not last longer than a minute. Nothing is more dangerous than to remain exposed to the open air, particularly if the room is not warm.

"In washing the whole body," said Father Kneipp, "begin either at the upper or the lower part, only be quick about it and *do not rub the skin dry*. The chief point is that the whole body should be wet and the water pressed gently into the pores. One should go over the same place three or four times with the sponge or the towel, which should be wet but not dripping so that the water may be well pressed in. As soon as the ablution is over the clothes must be put on rapidly and the warmth of the body preserved by at once taking exercise. If the patient gets out of bed to take this form of washing, he must go back to bed as soon as it is accomplished."

Many objected to not drying the body, but Father Kneipp insisted: "My method of not rubbing and drying the skin is by far the best. The water taken in by the pores quickly becomes warm and conveys its warmth to the skin. This produces rapid evaporation which taken up by the clothes develops an agreeable sensation of comfort to the whole body..."

For the partial washing, one proceeds in the same way as for the entire ablution. Father Kneipp explained the benefits of these washings as follows:

"Ablutions, whether entire or partial, develop easily an increase of warmth on the skin which penetrates deeper into the body...

"Cold water strengthens and fortifies. We will suppose a man to have been hard at work all day and his hands and feet weary and tired. He puts them for three or four minutes in cold water, the weariness disappears and strength comes back to them. This is the way cold water acts; it refreshes and strengthens the whole body...

"Both the entire and partial ablutions are so beneficial that many illnesses are quite cured by them alone. One or two instances will make this clear. The much-feared Influenza which is spreading far and wide ... may be quite cured by washings. If the patient will get out of bed every hour and take an entire washing rapidly, and at once get into bed again, and repeat this eight or 10 times, nay even 12, profuse perspiration will result, the dry skin and fever will disappear and the patient will be free of the malady. No other remedy will be necessary. Very severe colds or catarrhs may be cured in this simple way."

It was said many illnesses were quite cured by this liquid alone.

GOUT RELIEVED!

A woman was suffering from so-called wandering gout. Father Kneipp advised her every night to get out of bed and take an entire washing and get back into bed. Not only was she quite cured of the gout but her general health was greatly improved, said Father Kneipp. She could not speak too highly of this method.

SWOLLEN FEET AND DIFFICULT
BREATHING RELIEVED!

Another woman, named Martha, 48 years old, suffered every night from swollen feet and difficult breathing, causing her great discomfort. Father Kneipp ordered her to take an entire washing daily. At the end of three months, she said her feet were in the best possible condition, her breathing easier, her appetite improved, she could sleep better and she was quite free from flatulence which had formerly troubled her.

FOOT SORES DISAPPEARED!

Another case was that of a servant girl who for months had suffered with sores on the feet. It was only with great pain that she could perform her duties. Father Kneipp told her to take an entire washing every night, to get out of bed to take it, and return to bed as quickly as possible. She was to bind on the sores a cloth dipped in a decoction of shave-grass. In about 10 weeks, the feet were all healed, and the girl's health, as she expressed it, better than ever.

SKIN ERUPTIONS VANISHED!

A woman named Christina complained that she often had eruptions on various parts of her body, and had taken many kinds of medicine in vain. Father Kneipp advised her to take an entire washing three times a week, either when she woke up in the night or when she rose in the morning. She followed this advice, and in the course of a few weeks, he says, was completely cured.

HEADACHES GONE!

A woman named Johanna suffered incessantly from intense headaches which were looked upon as incurable. Father Kneipp advised her to wade in water (up to her knees) once or twice a day, for the space of three or four minutes, and to take an entire washing three or four times a week, getting out of bed for this, and returning to bed afterward. Before a month had passed, she experienced great relief. "I was not at all surprised," said Father Kneipp. "The wading in water had drawn the blood down from the head and the washing had braced the whole body."

AMAZING RESULTS CLAIMED!

"How many thousands of people suffer from blood obstruction!" said Father Kneipp. "The blood does not flow regularly through the veins! To get the circulation into perfect order, use the entire washing three or four times a week ... As a rule, the entire washing answers every purpose."[1]

FATHER KNEIPP'S FAMOUS HEALING BATHS!

"On going into a well-stocked chemist's shop we cannot help saying as we look around, 'Surely there are remedies enough here and to spare to relieve, if not to cure, every disease to which man is subject," said Father Kneipp.

"If I, on the other hand, declare water and herbs only to be my stock in trade for the healing and relieving of all human maladies, the thought may occur to many, 'This chemist with his two simple remedies is really too insignificant to deal with the large number of diseases and infirmities.' Yet pause for a moment! Just as one can make many garments out of one large bale of cloth, so we can obtain from water a number and variety of remedies not inferior to those in the well-stocked chemist's shop.

"There are many kinds of douches, which, if wisely combined and applied, have very special results on the body. Each

---

[1]"I must make one remark about the 'Ganzwaschung' or entire washing," said Father Kneipp. "To take one every day is not advisable; the body gets too much accustomed to it and therefore does not derive so much benefit from it. Many have told me that it is their habit to take one daily, and I have dissuaded them, believing they would derive more benefit if they took only two a week and on other days only half washings and wading in water. If the entire washing is prescribed for an illness, it must be continued as long as the illness remains and afterwards only every third or fourth day."

application has its own special name and use just as each jar in the chemist's shop is labelled with its contents."

The Eye Bath

The eye bath is simple and easy to take. "Having poured cold water into a basin, the forehead and eyes must be dipped in sufficiently far to cover the (eyes) which must be kept open while in the water," said Father Kneipp. "This will at first cause pain which will be overcome by perseverance; for water never causes harm. Keep the eyes in the water for four or five seconds, then lift them out and wink repeatedly so that they may be cleansed by the eye-lids. After a minute repeat the whole process and then again the third time and the good effects will soon appear. The eye-bath strengthens and purifies; and if there is any impure matter in the eyes, the water will disperse it. One may take an eye-bath with advantage every day, and it will hurt no more than washing the face.

"One sees the enormous benefit to the eye-bath when used for inflammation of the eyes from six to 12 times a day. Occasionally after applying this bath inflammation makes its appearance and may be regarded by some as the outcome of the eye-bath; but the case is quite otherwise. The effect of the eye-bath is to dissolve and disperse, and, should there be impure matter in the head, it is drawn out by its means through the eyes which become inflamed, if the matter is acid...

"An eye-bath can be made by mixing herbs in water—for example, make a light decoction of shave grass, or wormwood, fennel and eye-bright, or a good bath may be made of the green inner bark of the elder-tree. These are made use of in the same way as the simple eye-bath. When it is not possible for the patient to get these herbs, let him persevere with the simple eye-bath and all will come right. It is a good plan to change the eye-baths; one day a simple water bath, another day one of herbs...

"Eye-baths are so harmless that they may be taken without fear for all weaknesses of the eye. Whether the eyes be weak from overwork or as the result of an illness they may alike be strengthened by the use of the eye-bath..."

The Arm Bath

A priest was stung in the hand by an insect. The spot began to burn and be painful and the whole arm was so swollen that he feared blood-poisoning. In such a case as this, said Father Kneipp, nothing is better than a warm arm bath with hay-flowers in the water—it is powerful in drawing out the poisonous matter. The priest used this liquid, hot water, to bathe the arm and then applied wet compresses of water-soaked hayflowers. These he kept on for half an hour. A short time after, he repeated the process, and continued it for an hour. The pain gradually disappeared and the poison was drained out leaving its trace only in a red mark. This simple liquid, water, can provide amazing help for skin and hair.

"When in paralysis the arm becomes powerless through want of blood and warmth," said Father Kneipp, "plunge it into a warm bath for half an hour or even an hour and there will be no doubt of the success of the remedy. The strictest attention must be given to the necessity of taking a cold arm bath after every second or third warm one in order to give strength to the system.

"When gout attacks the joints of the hands or arms, the warm bath is an admirable means of relief. It may be taken two or three times a day, if a cold one is employed alternately, lasting from two to four minutes.

"Abscesses and whitlows are easily cured by arm-baths of hayflowers in cold water and wet bandages. If the hand has been swollen for a long time by rheumatism or if the swellings have become hard, douches will be of the greatest service and an arm bath now and then will accelerate the cure..."

The Foot Bath

"Even as a boy," recalled Father Kneipp, "I noticed how country people took foot baths both warm and cold. They were constantly ordered by physicians for various illnesses ... It used to be a common practice among country people in summer, when they had finished their day's work, to sit outside the house and rest while at the same time, they put their feet in a pan of cold water for a few minutes. They declared it took away their tiredness and freshened them up as much as a good night's rest

... Formerly the people, especially the old and feeble, took cold foot baths in summer and warm in winter...

"As regards the length of time the feet should be in the water, my opinion is that it should never exceed a quarter of an hour: the doctors whom I have known and who recommend these baths give 14 minutes as the outside limit. I constantly recommend warm foot baths and my experience tells me that the time fixed by the doctors is best. But I give more cold than warm ... as a rule the feet should not remain in a cold bath longer than three or four minutes ... On first putting the feet into water, a sharp sensation of cold will be felt which will gradually pass and be followed by an agreeable sensation of warmth (this cycle is felt two or three times, and when the water itself feels warm, the bath should end)..."

The use of the cold foot bath is to draw the blood downward, said Father Kneipp. This liquid is excellent for relief of kidney, bladder, and urinary difficulties, he said. "If the footbath is taken wisely, that is, for a short time only, and exercise taken immediately after it, so that the feet get thoroughly warm," said Father Kneipp, there is no remedy so good for urinary troubles. (If the feet cannot be warmed by this method, it is best to take a warm foot bath.)

"To those who suffer from weak voice or ... loss of voice the cold foot bath cannot be too highly recommended. It is equally good for those who suffer from constipation and blood obstruction in the lower part of the body and is of special benefit to women...

"The warm foot bath works in much the same way as the cold. It is generally prescribed for old people ... The warm bath comforts old people and if taken for about a quarter of an hour (or rather less) in the evening, they nearly always fall asleep after it ... put oat-straw, hay-flower and other herbs into the water (hay-flower is best). These baths, taken for 14 minutes, will develop warmth, conduct the blood downward, and strengthen the feet. Baths, with these additions, should always be taken warm.

"Oat-straw and hay-flower foot baths are of the greatest service in gout, severe colds and weak or perspiring feet; also in urinary troubles, blood obstructions, diseased bones, especially where they are injured by overwork and strained and consequently brittle; they are also very good in cases of abscesses of bones and muscles..."

The Sitting Bath

A farmer caught a severe cold by getting wet through. He was unable to pass urine, and suffered intense pain. Father Kneipp ordered him to take a warm sitting bath for four or five minutes. It warmed the lower part of his body, the cramp disappeared, and with it the difficulty of passing urine.

"As a severe cold can be suppressed by a warm bath, so great heat in the lower part of the body may be removed by a cold sitting bath," said Father Kneipp. "I give an example. A man suffered greatly from piles. When he became overheated by work and much walking, his pain and trouble were almost unbearable, and in addition to this the heat flew to his head giving him violent pain. A cold sitting bath cooled the abdomen and brought him great relief. Now comes the question, 'How often can such a sitting bath, be taken?'

Bowel Pain Relieved

"A gentleman told me that the sitting bath had afforded him great relief from pain in, and constipation of, the bowels and consequently he made use of it constantly. The result was that he began to get a good deal of pain and to lose daily much blood. The frequent sitting baths had conducted too much blood downward; this clotted and produced piles by straining the blood vessels of the rectum.

"I am in favor of sitting baths if taken in moderation ... In cases of great heat or inflammation of the bowels I give a cold sitting bath once or twice in the week, sometimes thrice, but never oftener. If more be necessary, then a half bath is preferable...

"I invariably, when using the warm sitting bath, mix shave grass, oat-straw and young pinewood, or salt, in the water as I am convinced of their efficacy. Sitting baths are good if not used too often..."

The Half Bath

The half bath reaches up to the chest. "I never permit it longer than from two to six seconds," said Father Kneipp. "Using the half bath beyond the time ordered takes so much warmth from the body that it is difficult to reinstate it ... The results of the half bath are excellent; it braces and strengthens the body, develops heat, has a greater influence on the circulation of the

blood than any other application and helps greatly to con-
valescence after severe illness ... the shorter the time the better
... it is wiser to take two short baths than one long one ... The
baths must be taken while the patient is quite warm and
exercise must follow immediately after to promote natural
warmth (even if you already feel warm) ... Those patients who
are unable to take exercise after bathing should at once go to bed
and, where possible, a warm bed...

"The half bath is efficacious in many diseases, in relaxed or
inactive condition of the bowels and in cases of general weakness
... It must not be thought, however, that because the influence of
the half bath upon the body is so excellent, therefore, it must be
taken constantly ... Too much is injurious. A gentleman who
had derived great benefit from the use of the half bath took it for
a longer period each day and some days took it twice. As time
went on he found that gradually he was losing strength and
energy, and the difficulty of getting back his normal warmth was
each week greater and he naturally became depressed. In fact,
his constitution could no longer bear the incessant attacks of the
cold water. I advised him to give up all application of water
entirely for three weeks and then only to take two half baths a
week of the shortest duration. This treatment succeeded in
bringing back his natural warmth, strength and good spirits..."

The Cold Full Bath

"Of all baths the full bath is the most powerful," said Father
Kneipp. "Every part of the body, except the head, is under water.
It is well to take from four to six seconds to step in and get
thoroughly covered. There should be no hurry. The length of
time to remain is as a rule one or two seconds, or four or five
seconds ... Just as it is necessary to be quite warm in stepping
into the bath, so it is equally necessary to dress immediately...

"A general cry was raised at my demand that the body
should not be dried after a bath but the clothing at once put on.
My reason for this is that the warmth is greater and that it
comes more quickly if the clothes are put on rapidly and the
drying omitted ... the person is perfectly free from damp before
he has finished dressing. Nor does one feel damp, for the reason
that all is quickly converted into a warm steam which produces
an agreeable glow to the skin ... I require the person to walk or
work. By this he gets back more quickly his natural warmth (if

chill returns you must exercise again) ... It sometimes happens to one who has taken a full bath in the morning or at midday that towards evening his feet are very stiff and heavy ... Such a condition is not rare after taking the bath and comes about in this way. A man feels tolerably warm after the bath and cuts short the exercise, the warmth does not last and the feet cannot perspire. The weariness and heaviness are easily removed by wading a minute or two in water or walking on wet earth or wet stones (or bind a wet cloth around the feet at bedtime, and the stiffness will soon disappear)...

"During the last five years I have made many experiments with cold water and I am convinced that in almost every case the cold water is the reliable remedy. If on occasion it should be necessary to use a warm application in order to reinstate the normal warmth I think it can be done better by means of compresses than warm baths. There have been many thousands of patients here this year, and yet I have not ordered a single warm bath ... What cannot be effected with cold water cannot be effected with warm. The latter is useful as a side help in combination with cold baths, but warm baths alone never heal nor cure a disease...

"I know that warm baths are much used in rheumatism of the joints and in gout, but I never guaranteed a cure by their means, because I am sure that both these diseases are more easily and more effectively got rid of by cold douches and baths than by warm ones.

"This statement of mine has been disputed with some show of reason by those who have experienced the power of warm water to dissolve and disperse evil matter in rheumatism and gout, but even acknowledging the truth of this I still maintain my opinion, because my experience has taught me that the warm baths weaken the body, that the mischief they have removed comes back almost immediately with increased force. The system has no longer the power to resist; a little cold or trifling neglect will bring all the pain and sorrow back. On the other hand when the cure has been effected by cold water the body is so braced and strengthened that the cure is permanent.

"As regards herbs in the baths I have nothing but praise. I prefer hay-flowers, oat-straws and pine-shoots, and for diseases of the bladder such as gravel or stone there is nothing better than baths of oat-straw. I strongly recommend those who suffer from these to take one or two oat-straw baths in a month, at first warm and of 10 minutes' duration; then cold for five or six seconds; then again warm. Two or three of these will bring relief to the sufferer."

THE DOUCHES

"If a tree is to be removed from the earth," said Father Kneipp, "the attack must first be made on the roots ... Exactly so is it with diseases embedded in our system ... If therefore the sick place only be operated on, the roots of the tree of sickness will remain in the system and the sick person will never be well...

"I am convinced that there is no disease which does not gradually make itself felt throughout the whole body (even when it is only a sore finger or toe) ... therefore it is my firm opinion that those methods of healing are best which support, strengthen and brace up the whole body, thereby enabling it to throw off all hurtful matter and to resist any development of disease within it...

"I once met a gardener, well known to me in Augsburg, who was full of trouble and complained to me that the doctors had decided to amputate two of the fingers of his right hand and that the operation was to take place in two days. Up to his sixtieth year this man was fat, strong and healthy; he now looked wretched and ill, he had lost weight and his whole appearance was one of suffering; he had lost all his brightness and good humor by the pain and sickness he had gone through. The hand was frightful to look at; it was so swollen that it was impossible to say whether it was one malignant ulcer or whether there were any fingers at all. As the man so bitterly grieved over and feared the coming operation, I advised him as a last resort to try the water cure. This he was ready and glad to do. The effect of the water upon the body and upon the fingers was to take away the intense pain and the whole hand suffered less.

"Every application brought relief, so that the excellent effects of the water applications on the body and on the hand in a short time were very remarkable. He made up his mind not to allow his fingers to be taken off and at the same time persevered with the water applications until at length the hand was healed leaving only little scars, and he was able to use the hand as well as ever. The application of water to the whole body strengthened it in its effort to cast out the diseased matter, and the benefit to the arm in dissolving and dispersing corrupt elements was equally great. Gradually the whole body became healthy. This is what I call healing.

"The cure of all diseases should be undertaken in the same way as in the example I have just given. The whole body must be treated and in this way the diseased part will be healed. These reasons have induced me regularly to work upon the whole organism; at the same time, however, in order not to act upon it too severely, I treat from time to time a special part of it and then again another. In very severe cases of illness I have found the simple washings with water ineffectual, and have therefore had recourse to douches which have answered extremely well on the various parts of the body. As each special douche exercised its influence on a particular part, a combination of them was made use of for the whole body."

The Head Douche

The head douche is applied by beginning on the right or left side, or behind the ear and continuing to the middle of the head. From this point the water must flow quite evenly over the whole head. One can of water is generally sufficient. Just as a tired hand gains strength by washing it in cold water, so the head loses weariness and gains strength by using the head douche, said Father Kneipp. It should not be given too often, for if it were, too much blood would be conducted to the head, and repeated wetting would probably produce neuralgia.

The Face Douche

The face douche consists simply of douching the whole face in the same way that the head was douched. It is employed in the cure of ulcers, Lupus and other skin diseases which attack the face, said Father Kneipp. The water must be confined only to the face.

The Ear Douche

The ear douche is useful in cases of deafness, said Father Kneipp. The person bows his head, as for the upper douche (see page 277) and the water is poured from the water can on one side of the head round about the ear and then on the other in the same way. The water is not poured into the ear, but if by chance some finds its way in it will not matter, said Father Kneipp. Two cans of water may be used for the ear douche. After the ear douche the head should be well covered until quite dry, unless the temperature of the room is warm, in which case it will not be necessary. There is no objection to going into the fresh air after it, if the weather is warm and there is no wind, said Father Kneipp.

The effect of this douche is to strengthen and remove blood obstructions and disperse foul secretions, he said. It is very strengthening. If one is very careful, it may be taken three, four and even five times a week with very good results. Its action will not be on the ear alone but on every part of the head, particularly where blood obstructions exist.

The Breast Douche

This is usually taken in combination with the upper douche. The patient bends one arm upward and leans on the other, which renders easy the pouring of the water on the chest from the side. At Father Kneipp's health spa, those who took this douche usually lay on their back on a board, to get a good strong douche on the breast. This douche is strengthening and dissolving, said Father Kneipp. It loosens the mucus in the chest and makes its discharge easy. It is absolutely necessary that the heart be strong and in perfect order for a person to take the breast douche, said Father Kneipp.

The Arm Douche

The arm douche consists of douching the whole arm, beginning with the fingers (every one of which must be douched) and continuing up to the shoulder. The whole process must not take more than a minute. "It is generally employed when powerlessness of the arm sets in, caused either by paralysis or any like trouble," said Father Kneipp, "or when the arm is very feeble and abnormally cold, or in rheumatism of the arm. In writer's cramp and neuralgia generally it is a most excellent remedy." It may be taken every day and in exceptional cases twice a day. Just as the feet are strengthened by the knee douche, so the arm may be made quite strong by applications of cold water from time to time, said Father Kneipp.

The Upper Douche

"In administering an upper douche," said Father Kneipp, "one must take into consideration the parts of the body which will be subject to its action. These are the heart, the lungs, the bronchial tubes and the vocal chords. This being so, one must be advised whether the douche is to be weak or strong or even at first whether it may be given at all. For example, in case of lung disease it would not be wise to begin with the upper douche, but to substitute for a time washing the upper part of the body morning and evening with cold water and to increase the action by mixing vinegar with the water. I advise the same for one who has palpitation or any other disease of the heart; otherwise, it may be safely administered in all cases ... Should a few days' trial of the upper washing prove a success, then the upper douche may follow, which will gradually strengthen the patient. This advice must be strictly followed in heart problems..."

An upper douche is given, beginning from the neck down one half the back. The water, which may be given from a hose or a water can, should spread evenly like a sheet over the back. (Father Kneipp preferred a watering can, because with it the stream can be more easily regulated, and increased or diminished at will.) Where patients have taken several douches and with them have made great progress, three or four cans may be used, he said, and for a very hardy person, even six, seven or eight. "If a sick person bears the upper douche well, its power may be gradually increased," said Father Kneipp. "If the upper part of the body is weak, one begins gently with the left or right arm, coming gradually from one side to the other with the water till the loins are reached."

Before taking an upper douche, the upper part of the body should be quite warm, said Father Kneipp. As soon as it is over, a shirt or chemise must go on as quickly as possible, followed by the remaining articles of clothing, without drying the body at all. After the body is covered, the neck and hair, if they have become wet, should be made dry, and exercise should be taken until the whole body has recovered its normal warmth.

The Hip Douche

This is a continuation of the knee douche (see page 279), and exercises its influence particularly upon the kidneys, the liver and bladder and upon all parts of the abdomen, said Father

Kneipp. It regulates the blood in the lower part of the body and has great curative power in case of piles.

To give a hip douche, take either a water can or hose and begin to pour the water at the back part of the feet and bring it up very slowly and gradually till the knee is reached; then over the hip halfway to the back. "With beginners," said Father Kneipp, "one always commences from the feet, gradually getting the stream higher—one does it in the same way with people who suffer from continuous cold feet in order that the blood should rapidly find its way to them, for where the water first falls that part is the soonest warmed. We say emphatically that douching from below to above must be conducted very slowly. If it is begun at the hip, douche first one and then the other rapidly, and this may be done three or four times, we repeat here that the water must flow equally over the hip so that it looks as though covered with a sheet of glass...

"When four or five douches have been taken from the feet upward there is no harm in beginning from the hip because the blood is now in better order. Those which strengthen the most are those which are given from the upper part of the hip, the water flowing to the feet. For the hip douche one uses from six to 10 cans full of water containing about 4 gallons. For a weak person one canful is enough at first, then later two or three, and if the effect of these is good the amount can be increased. If the body is in good condition and able to bear the action of these douches on the abdomen, three or four cans of water may be used, and in cases where special force is required five or six cans..."

Father Kneipp recommended this liquid—in the form of hip douches—as beyond comparison the best for acting upon the kidneys. Its effect is not only to strengthen but to dissolve and disperse, he said. It is also excellent for the bladder, liver and all abdominal organs, and will relieve headaches.

"While the knee douche acts beneficially upon part of the abdomen as well as upon the feet, so the hip douche benefits *all* parts of the abdomen," said Father Kneipp.

"A girl suffered so much from headache that she was compelled to keep to her bed, and every remedy she applied seemed to increase the suffering. In order to free her from pain, I prescribed a powerful hip douche, the result being that in a short time the headache disappeared and she was able to get a few hours sleep. Evidently in this case the cause of the headache was stomach trouble and this being removed by the hip douche she obtained relief.

"A man named Jacob suffered intensely from cramp in the feet. I prescribed hip douches, back douches and half baths and by these he was completely cured, though I think the most effective were the hip douches. As the hip douche is easy to take and as the abdomen and indeed the whole system can bear it well, it may be taken two, three or four times a week, according to the strength of the patient."

The Knee Douche

This douche is applied from below to above the knee and is a reinforcement of the foot bath. One begins at the instep, covers the foot and continues the stream upward to above the knee. For weak people it will be enough at first to use one can of water for both knees while for those who are strong, two, three or four may be poured on, said Father Kneipp.

Like a strong foot bath, its special object is to attract the blood to the feet, to increase the normal warmth and to brace and strengthen the whole body. Those who suffer constantly from cold feet may take the knee douche two or three times a week, said Father Kneipp. It is of great benefit in urinary trouble, diseases of the stomach and kidney and in removing headaches which are caused by too much blood in the head, he said. Even sore throats are relieved by this douche because of its power to strengthen and draw the blood downward, he claimed.

The water must flow evenly and smoothly down over the foot, to hold in the warmth which would otherwise evaporate. This warmth is then increased under the water, all the more so in response to the coldness of the water. This is why the water should never be splashed on helter-skelter, but rather evenly and quietly. Otherwise, the body will indeed become cold.

The Back Douche

The back douche commences from below and is directed gradually upward till the water flows in a gentle, even stream over the shoulders, forming a sheet of water which spreads over half the back. When the water is poured from the middle of the back upwards, it does not matter which side is first douched, right or left, as long as the water flows quietly and uninterruptedly over the whole surface. When both sides have been douched, one can direct the water either up or down the middle of the back—the more quietly and uninterruptedly the water flows over the middle and both sides of the back the better. It is a great mistake when the back douche is turned into a spraying douche, and when the stream is poured on the back from a distance of a quarter or half a yard, or when the water is thrown superficially on the surface, said Father Kneipp.

"I know of no douche so generally strengthening as the back douche," said Father Kneipp. "Its effects are excellent. It is of the greatest service in regulating the circulation of the blood and in dissolving and dispersing obstructions in the blood and secretions. It braces and strengthens the lower part of the body, in that it disperses gases, and works upon the liver and kidneys; its effect is also very good upon the breast and indeed upon the whole body, which it warms and strengthens and purifies ... In most cases ... it must be taken in combination with other douches once or twice a week only and then only for a very short time."

The Full Douche

One does not take the full douche until the system is prepared for it by first taking the knee douche, the hip douche, the upper douche, the back douche and the half bath, said Father Kneipp. When all parts of the body have been prepared and strengthened, the full douche comes in with greatest benefit to the whole body. "The body must be thoroughly warm, and unless it be so, on no account must the douche be taken," said Father Kneipp. "The very best time to take it is in full perspiration."

One begins the full douche from the heels upward to the hips, then over the whole back to the shoulders, over which the water must flow backward and forward as evenly as possible over the whole body. Or one may begin at the shoulders, pouring the water first over the back and then over the front of the body. The water must flow evenly on both sides of the body, gently.

"It must not be supposed that spraying or wetting the body in all sorts of ways, whether with hose or water can, is a full douche," said Father Kneipp. It must be administered according to instructions or it is no full douche. When the body has been prepared by applications for the full douche, as many as eight or

10 cans of water may be used at one time. For a very weak person, one would begin with one or two cans of water, but as his or her strength increases, the person will not be content with less than eight or 10 and sometimes asks for 12, said Father Kneipp.

Another way to give a full douche is this. The patient kneels in a large bathtub and bends slightly forward. A very light full douche is then administered, and then comes the pail and the water is dashed over the entire body. When an invalid is so far improved as to be able to take a full douche, it is the best indication of renewed life, said Father Kneipp. The full douche is used in combination with other applications once or twice a week. It can be taken early in the morning or before the midday meal. If in the afternoon, it will be better to let two hours pass by after the meal. In taking the full douche it is better not to wet the head (if wet it must be rubbed thoroughly dry).

The Lightning Douche

To give the lightning douche correctly, one begins at the heel of the right foot and works slowly upwards till the whole back is douched, and this process is repeated for the front of the body. In the meantime, a comfortable heat is developed and the sick person is so relieved that he says, "I feel newborn," says Father Kneipp. If you wish to know something of the effect of the lightning douche, go and look at a burning building. In order to quench the flames, a hose is directed to them with such force that the burning wall sometimes caves in.

In the same way, through a hose, the water is directed like lightning over the body, beginning either from above or below. This lightning-like stream, although it takes a good strong hold, is by no means painful, but, said Father Kneipp, it drives out everything from the system that is impure or harmful.

In giving the lightning douche, the distance of the hose from the patient is from 3 to 5 yards, according to the force desired for the jet, and the application may last from three to eight minutes. First a full, sharp douche is given, then the finger is placed across the opening so that the stream is broken and a rapid spray dashes against the body like a rainstorm against a window. The effects of the lightning douche are as follows, said Father Kneipp: "Increased warmth, improved appearance, lighter breathing, better appetite, free expectoration, and unusual amount of and deposit in the urine, at which last symptom many are needlessly alarmed." According to the condition of the patient, the lightning douche may be applied every second day, every day or even twice a day, he said.

A young priest who, on account of disease of the heart (weak valve) could not advance in his profession, used this simple, natural liquid in lightning douches. The first day before taking the douche, his pulse was 108—after it, it was not more than 80. He felt extremely well and declared: "There is nothing the matter with me; I have not felt so well and comfortable for years."

FATHER KNEIPP'S FAMOUS HOME CURES FOR GRIEVOUS AILMENTS!

Asthma

"As this illness is caused by the impure, watery and slimy blood and by the corrupt state of the lungs, and indeed of the whole system, there is no difficulty in dealing with it both outwardly and inwardly," said Father Kneipp.

"If the sufferer can lie down, place on his chest a six-fold cloth previously dipped in hot water and vinegar as warm as he can bear it, it will not be long before the cramp disappears. Should one application not suffice, or if the cloth cools too soon, replace it by another at the end of 15 or 20 minutes. If the cramp yields to the treatment the cloth may be removed; otherwise, the great heat of the blood would clog the chest ... If the patient cannot lie down, lay the cloth dipped in hot water and vinegar on the stomach, or instead of this a warm bag containing soaked hay-flowers. As soon as artificial warmth is generated in the stomach, it spreads to the chest and diverts the blood down-wards, making the pain more bearable and eventually removing it. Should the first attack pass off, a second may be looked for with certainty; therefore, the applications to the stomach must be renewed as soon as the natural warmth decreases to prevent, if possible, a return of the pain...

"For warming and especially for quieting the cramp the most suitable thing is tea made of silver weed, camomile and mint. Milk with fennel boiled in it and drunk as hot as possible is also an excellent remedy for an attack of cramp. For the improvement of the gastric juices and the promotion of digestion

I can strongly recommend a spoonful every hour of tea made of wormwood, juniper berries, shave-grass and angelica. The wormwood strengthens and helps the stomach, the angelica carries off bad matter, the shave-grass purifies and juniper berries empty it of slime." In less than a month, the asthma should be gone, with these applications and remedies, said Father Kneipp.

Reported Cases:

- A gentleman from Hungary had suffered from asthma for many years. It had gotten so bad in recent months that he could not sleep and felt he was suffocating. Father Kneipp at once ordered that his back be dry-rubbed. This was immediately followed by an upper douche, a knee douche and exercise. The next morning, the man joyfully reported that he had slept well for the first time in years. He took an upper and a back douche, and soaked in water for two minutes—and the second night passed well. This treatment was continued for three weeks: one day an upper and a hip douche, another day an upper douche and a hip bath, on another a knee douche and back douche. Internally, he took wormwood, shave-grass and juniper berries boiled together. This carried off a good deal of bad matter in the urine. He gained a better appetite and looked younger. In four weeks, he was quite cured.

- A professor said he had suffered for many years from attacks of asthma, and often could not work. During a severe attack, he was given a compress of this amazing liquid (a cloth dipped in hot water and vinegar laid on his chest as hot as he could stand it). In 20 minutes, the attack was over and the patient felt quite comfortable. After this, he was told to get out of bed twice daily and wash completely. Applications of water and vinegar were renewed four or five times. Then the attacks returned, and Father Kneipp switched the hot cloth to the man's stomach, causing the blood to be drawn downward, away from the lungs, and the chest was relieved. Next, the hot cloth was placed over the man's feet and legs. In this way, the blood was directed to the feet and the chest still further relieved. "Thus treated," says Father Kneipp, "the blood was gradually brought into proper circulation. When needful, hot water was used, but when cold water bandages supplied the necessary warmth the hot water applications were dispensed with." In three weeks, the man was normal.

Eyesight Restored!

"The eyes can be strengthened," said Father Kneipp, "by eye baths, by holding them once, twice or even thrice from two to five seconds in water, winking and then lifting the head out of the water to immerse it again a few seconds after; this process should be repeated three or four times, the whole lasting about a minute. Such baths cleanse and strengthen the eyes and can be strongly recommended not only when the eyes are bad but even when in good condition. In addition to these so-called eye baths, eye bandages or applications are recommended.

"Take a small piece of linen folded five or six times, dip it in cold water and then bind it over the eyes; leave it there four or five minutes and then repeat the process. This simple bandage has a wonderfully strengthening effect upon the eyes. Instead of water bandages, herb bandages may be used with equal advantage for cleansing and strengthening the eyes. Put a teaspoonful of powdered fennel into a quart of water, boil it and strain it, then dip the rag into it and lay it on quite wet; the liquid should penetrate the eye.

"If a rag be dipped in wormwood tea and laid on the eyes in the same way, the effect is almost equally beneficial. These herbs cleanse and strengthen the eyes. Other ingredients may be used with advantage, for example, aloes, shave-grass and alum, the last, however, very much diluted ... Just as one extinguishes an outburst of fire with water, so may you drive inflammation of the eyes away by the same means ... Eye water may be made from honey; a teaspoonful of honey is boiled in a quart of water for four or five minutes and furnishes a good eye bath. The honey purifies and strengthens, decreases the heat and relieves pain...

"I have never had any difficulty in clearing up cloudy or filmy eyes ... We have many means of removing these clouds from the eyes. A very greatly diluted alum water[2] is beneficial. Still I do not confine myself to the use of it for long, but make use of other dispersing remedies as well. A drop of honey daily and twice a day washing the eyes with alum water have a dispersing and healing effect...

---

[2]Father Kneipp said that alum water may be made by placing a small portion of alum on the point of a knife in a half cup of water. It should be taken in the same way as a simple eye bath, he said, but not too often. He also used water in combination with other Rapid Healing Foods.

"For example, a girl came to me a short time ago who could scarcely see at all (she had a film over her eyes). With this method, it was not long before the film was entirely removed and the girl saw as clearly as before...

"Fennel water is specially good; it so strengthens the eye as to make the sight clearer. Eye bandages are very good in their effect; a very soft, washed-out piece of linen is dipped in aloe water and laid on for a couple of hours, renewed, however, every half hour; one may also be applied at night. If the eye is still easily inflamed, then use wormwood water either for washing or bandaging the eye. Wormwood and tormentilla sugar produces a special effect in cases of outbreaks on the eyes.

"Extract of tormentilla or wormwood is mixed with white sugar, stirred together and set out in the open air; the spirit quickly evaporates while the sugar dries and retains the essential parts of the wormwood and tormentilla and may be applied to the eyes once or twice daily. If the sugar be not too fine it gives a gentle friction when blown into the eye and greatly facilitates the disperson of the clouds. The sugar, however, rapidly vanishes and sugar water mingled with dispersed matter flows from the eyes..."

Cataract

"Cataract is considered by the profession in general as incurable except by an operation," said Father Kneipp. "Nevertheless I am of the opinion that help may be afforded without this, if taken in time. Many patients have been aided by me not only at the commencement of the formation of cataract but even when further advanced. In such cases I have found it needful to include the whole body in the process of dissolving and dispersing and not to confine myself to the eyes only.

"Bandages are, for instance, employed in stronger forms than usual; those suffering from cataract should take two or three head douches weekly and one or two neck rollers or swathing bands, as well as one or two eye baths daily in addition to the use of eye salve (honey mixed with green herbs). I need hardly say that the greatest prudence must be exercised in the use of all these..."

Gutta Serena or Amaurosis

"This form of blindness consists in the gradual dying away of the visual nerve. I have cured partially blind cases of Gutta

Serena as well as some quite blind," said Father Kneipp. "For example, a Pole had been quite blind for three years and in three weeks he was cured, and so with several in whom the mischief had not been of long standing. It is of great importance in curing this form of eye disease that one operates vigorously and that the interchange of matter should be promoted in the whole body as well as in the eyes, for I am convinced that in such eye diseases the entire body is sick.

"The strongest applications, if used with care, are here the most effectual; each day two or three eye baths, and weekly two or three head douches and two hip baths should be taken. These have a strengthening effect on the whole body as well as a dissolving and purifying one. I was especially successful with this disease when nicotine poisoning was the cause of it."

Glaucoma

"I have relieved glaucoma with great success," said Father Kneipp. "To cure glaucoma, it is essential in the first place that all superfluous blood-currents be drawn off from the head and by rapid interchange of matter, the obstruction gradually decreased so that the eyes may once more attain to their former strength.

"In glaucoma, each delay is fraught with the greatest danger. In treating it one operates less on the head than on the whole body, for strong measures applied to the head would only direct more blood to it. It will be sufficient to take frequent eye baths and provide for the purifying and strengthening of the eyes by the remedies already given.[3]

"Above all, an endeavor must be made to bring the circulation of the blood into order; as a rule, people suffering from glaucoma generally have ... too much blood in the upper part of the body." The following cure is described:

"A theologian was suffering from glaucoma and could no longer see to read. He was ordered to walk daily in water for the purpose of diverting the blood from the head, also to take three hip baths every week in order to warm and strengthen the abdomen and further two complete douches to regulate the

---

[3]Glaucoma can result in permanent blindness. Glaucoma victims are warned not to self-treat without a doctor's approval. As with all ailments described in this book, you are advised to seek a doctor's help immediately. This material is presented for information only. Self-treatment is not recommended.

circulation of the blood. Beyond all this, he took two eye baths daily and washed his eyes with wormwood tea alternately with the aloe water.

"The best means of drawing the blood from the head are foot baths and thigh and knee douches. Strong people may take upper douches, but weak people must be content with washing the upper part of the body.

"If glaucoma makes its appearance suddenly ... in such case it is best to take what is called a short bandage or if the invalid be strong enough a Spanish mantle," said Father Kneipp. These, he said, are taken as follows:

1. *Short Bandage:* First lay a blanket on the bed and on this a cloth which is to be used as the bandage. It must be at least four-fold and of rough linen. It must have been dipped in water and partially wrung out to prevent dripping. On this the patient lies while the cloth goes well up to the arms and down to the knees; it is then folded closely over the body so as to adhere to the skin in every part and to exclude the air, the two ends being laid carefully over each other. The blanket, which should extend above and below the bandage, is brought round so as completely to wrap the body within it. Remove after a half hour. Take gentle exercise or stay in bed for an hour and get some sleep.

2. *Spanish Mantle:* This bandage or mantle is really a long shirt or chemise reaching below the feet, which has been soaked in water and wrung out. A blanket is laid on the bed, upon which the patient, wrapped in his Spanish mantle, places himself. The blanket is then brought together about his body, snugly, and kept on from an hour and a half to two hours, says Father Kneipp.

"One may also envelop the feet as high as the calves in a cloth which has been dipped in water and vinegar, half of each, but at most only for an hour," said Father Kneipp. "After three days the blood will be drawn off from the head, and then alternate knee and thigh douches and hip baths can be used. These must be used in moderation; two applications daily are quite enough."

Skin Diseases

"If the blood be good," said Father Kneipp, "the condition of the individual is also good; if the blood be bad, that is to say, mixed with impure matter, the whole body suffers for it. When, therefore, a part of the body is attacked with eruptions, there flows through the afflicted part the same blood as through the other portions of the body, and the part attacked by eruptions is merely the point which nature itself has chosen as the exit for the evil matter.

"In order to effect a cure here, not only should the part of the body on which the eruption appears be treated, but the whole body must be operated upon in order to draw off and expel all the evil matter. This is best done by supplying the patient with good nourishment which forms better blood.

"By applications of water a quicker change of matter takes place and the health is improved until by degrees all diseased matter is drawn off and expelled and the whole system strengthened."

As an example, Father Kneipp gives the case of a patient named Maria, who said, "My face is often full of pimples. Then they go away and come again, generally on my arms and feet but sometimes on other parts of the body. I have seen many doctors who have prescribed ointments for rubbing in, and sharp water for ablutions. For years I have used all sorts of remedies. Still the eruption has spread and my strength has gradually decreased, while my whole appearance is unhealthy."

Maria was ordered to wear a shirt dipped in hay-flower water twice a week for an hour or an hour and a half, and to wrap herself in a woolen cloth. She was also to take two half baths in the week for two seconds only, and as she was strong enough two complete douches were given her within the seven days.

The shirt not only softened the bad matter but drew it out of the body. The half baths strengthened the system and the complete shower baths induced great activity, generated warmth, as well as a general violent transpiration.

After six days the eruption was reduced to a gentle redness, and after 12 days the eruption entirely disappeared; then Maria was ordered the following applications: a wet shirt, two thigh douches, two hip baths and a complete shower bath, and having used these for two weeks, she was quite well. She acquired a splendid appetite, she slept well and her strength increased daily.

Internally she took daily, morning and evening, 3 to 4 spoonfuls of tea made of bark or oak, sage and wormwood.

Catarrh of the Bladder
(Inflammation)

Father Kneipp knew well the many symptoms of bladder inflammation—including heavy pressure, violent cramp, thick urine, frequent desire to urinate without result, infection and pus—which can last for years. He said the only cure is this amazing liquid to cleanse and purify the urinary organs, carry off the impure matter and build up the diseased organs. The best means of accomplishing this, he said, is by douches, bandages and hip baths. As an example, Father Kneipp gives the case of a patient named Augustine, who came to the priest with the following complaints:

> "I have suffered for many months from what the doctors call bladder inflammation. I have tried many remedies which have given me only temporary help, if indeed you can call it help at all. I am always wanting to make water without result. I often suffer from cramps, and the urine is generally cloudy and mixed with putrid pus and leaves a thick sediment behind. I am always thirsty, I have but little appetite, and feel weak."

Since he was otherwise in good condition, and his lungs, heart and liver were healthy, Father Kneipp prescribed this amazing liquid in douches, hip baths and teas. During the week he had three thigh douches, one back douche, three hip baths and two knee douches, and every morning and evening a washing of the upper part of the body. In addition to these, a four-fold cloth dipped in hay-flower water was laid on his stomach three times a week for an hour and a half each time. At the end of three-quarters of an hour, the cloth was dipped afresh and laid on. The first time the hay-flower water was warm, the second time cold. The hay-flower cloth dispelled, absorbed and operated upon the cause of the cramp. The thigh douches checked the heat, strengthened the system, softened the hardened matter and expelled all putrid stuff. The back douches operated in a strengthening way on the whole body. The hip baths were equally strengthening in their effect upon the body, besides moderating the heat, which had spread itself over the body.

After 10 days of treatment with this amazing liquid, Augustine reported that the heat had decreased, that large quantities of putrid matter were expelled, that the urine was improved, that the too-frequent desire to urinate had ceased, and that he felt much better. In order to continue this improvement, he was told to take three hip baths, two complete douches and a bandage (soaked in water) on the abdomen each week for two weeks. Again there was a great improvement. For the next four weeks, he had a third prescription: two hip baths, two complete douches, and frequent wading in water each week. At the end of this time, the water treatments were reduced by half.

At the end of six weeks, his condition was so changed that he could both sleep and eat well, he was much stronger and the urinary trouble was almost nonexistent. During the first two weeks of his treatment he took internally daily in two or three portions a cupful of tea made of dwarf-elder root, shave-grass and eight or 10 crushed juniper berries, all boiled together. The dwarf-elder root acted as a dissolvent and expellent, the shave-grass as a purifier and the juniper berries as a dispeller and purifier. The third and fourth week he took tea of oak-bark, wormwood and shave-grass. The oak-bark purifies, draws, and heals, while wormwood improves the gastric juices.

Instant Relief for
Complete Stoppage of Urine!

A day laborer caught a bad cold while digging a well. He got very wet, indeed soaked through, and suddenly experienced a severe chill in his whole body. He discovered that urine would pass only in drops and with great pain. Along with the chills, he developed a fever. A doctor's medicine did not help. Then he came to Father Kneipp, who promptly told him to use this amazing liquid in an abdominal vapor bath. Into a bed pan a handful of shave-grass was thrown and boiling water was poured on it. As quickly as possible, the patient sat on the stool so that the steam could operate thoroughly on the whole body.

He had not sat on the stool 20 minutes when he was able to pass large quantities of water, and the cramping pains soon ceased. "It seems almost unbelievable that such a painful ailment can be cured by such a simple remedy in so short a time, but seeing is believing," said this priest!

At the end of 20 minutes, the patient went to bed without washing himself so that the perspiration which had set in might last longer and disappear by degrees. After about two hours the sweating subsided, and the patient was washed with fresh water. This washing is very important, said Father Kneipp, as it protects the body from the cold air. Do not pour the water on. Simply wash.

The patient remained a day in bed undergoing two entire washings. A two-fold cloth was laid on the abdomen and also over the bladder and repeated as often as needed to get and maintain a normal temperature. Father Kneipp said that water mixed with vinegar has a very strengthening effect and normalizes temperature. The patient took nothing beyond tea of shave-grass and dwarf-elder root every two hours. He soon regained his appetite and was able to get back to his work.[4]

Diarrhea Relieved!

Father Kneipp's recommendations for relieving diarrhea were as follows: eat slowly, be moderate in drinking and especially avoid drinking while eating. To remove the diseased matter from the stomach and bowels, and strengthen the whole system, the best thing—he said—is a bandage on the stomach, which has been soaked in hay-flower water or water and vinegar. If you have a weak stomach, be sure the bandage or compress is warm. Later, when strength returns, he recommended vigorous applications of cold water "which can only bring health."

Reported Cases:

• A patient named Anna said: "Every two or three weeks I have diarrhea which makes me so weak and tired I can hardly work. I seldom have a good appetite and I don't dare eat much as it brings on diarrhea. I'm always thirsty and sleep very badly." Father Kneipp told her to lay a three-fold cloth previously dipped in hay-flower water on her abdomen, for an hour and a half, redipping it after 45 minutes, and to do this once a week. She was also told to

---

[4]Although further applications were not necessary—as a precaution—one or two complete washings were taken daily for a week. In a case like this, should the trouble return and one steam or vapor bath is not enough, a second may be taken, which, as a rule, is enough, said Father Kneipp. In extreme cases, the steaming and washing daily with vinegar and water has to be continued for three or four days. Such sufferers are usually overweight. When the steam is removed and the sweating has lasted two hours, the washing can be started. If sweat appears in washing, and little cramp pains return, the washing must be stopped and the steam repeated to relieve the pain.

take three times daily 3 spoonfuls of angelica root, wormwood and shave-grass tea. This tea empties the body of
poisons and improves digestion, he said. Every week, he
recommended two thigh douches, two half baths and a
back douche. "In this way," he says, "the whole system was
brought into better condition, the diseased matter was
carried off and the digestion was greatly improved."

● One man complained: "I suffered all last night with violent
diarrhea. I feel ill and exhausted and thirsty. What can I
do?" Father Kneipp advised him to boil some knot-grass in
half water and half red wine, and drink a cup of it, quite
warm. If the diarrhea continued he was to take a second
cup in two or three hours.[5] He was also told to dip a cloth in
hot water and vinegar and lay it on his abdomen for an
hour and a half renewing it after 45 minutes.

● A patient named Anthony said: "At every trifle I get
diarrhea. As soon as I get rid of it, it comes back. What can
I do?" Father Kneipp advised him to drink three times a
day 2 or 3 spoonfuls of tea made of oak-bark and wormwood and to take every second or third day a half bath, for
quick relief.

Diarrhea is easily cured, said Father Kneipp. To prevent its
recurrence, eat sensibly, avoid sudden changes of diet or overeating, eat good, wholesome, ripe fruit (not half ripe), avoid sweet
pastry and sugar. At the first sign of diarrhea, take a small cup
of tea made of centaury and wormwood, or tea made of sage and
camomile.

Swollen Feet

"Very often," said Father Kneipp, "swollen feet are the
result of faulty circulation. The blood is like a very sick man who
may have power to get a little way from home but not to get
back." In general, anything that increases circulation in the feet,
and throughout the body, will make swellings of the feet vanish,
he observed. It is quite easy to cure swollen feet, said Father
Kneipp.

● Swollen feet often occur after fevers and inflammations, if
the system has not been properly cleansed.

[5]Instead of knot-grass, wormwood and powdered fennel may be used,
making the tea the same way.

- Swollen feet are not unusual after erysipelas and scarlet fever, and attacks which usually have their origin in some kidney disease ... a kind of blood poisoning sets in.

- Swollen feet always occur to people who stand very much and who take very little exercise. "And yet help is so easy!" said Father Kneipp. "That which medicines cannot touch may be attained by water with the best results."

"How many have come to me, both men and women, having tightly bound their swollen feet in woolen bandages ... or elastic," said Father Kneipp. "Many of them had worn these bandages for two or three years running ... above the bandages on the legs and thighs bags were formed and the limbs were twice as big as they ought to be ... Without exception I ordered every person to remove their elastic or woolen bandages and the whole body to be promptly operated on (with washings) so as to expel the watery and sluggish matter within. In every case I was successful ... As a rule four to six weeks' treatment was sufficient to cleanse the system, using for the purpose only tea or herbs and applications of water. The patients soon recovered their appetite and healthy appearance and rejoiced in their renewed vigor.

"Although the bandages are bound to come off, yet I allow many to keep them on a few days longer, for when the system has too much matter in it which runs at once to the feet it would cause them to swell very much and this would take the spirit and courage of the patient away. So I first operate on the system internally and externally for the purpose of bracing and dispersing and then I order the bandages removed. As a rule no more swellings take place ... A proof of the correctness of my idea is furnished by those who, during the summer went barefoot and by those specially who had ulcers and open wounds on their feet ... the ulcers vanished ... the sores were an outlet for the foul matter...

"It was remarkable that those who had suffered year in and year out with cold feet soon got a good natural warmth into them. How many hundreds suffer; and how easily could they all be helped!"

A Reported Case:

"Every morning," said one man, "my feet swell and I am unable to walk. I feel like a cripple." Such a man is quite easily cured, said Father Kneipp, and this man was proof of it. In three weeks, he was so well that he said, "I feel like a new man. I cannot understand how in so short a time such a change could occur!"

"Now what brought this man's whole body into order again?" said Father Kneipp. "He took in the week three thigh douches, two back douches, two half baths and a complete douche, besides daily wading in water or having his knees douched with cold water. Further, he daily drank a cup of tea made of shave-grass, bark of oak and wormwood; the shave-grass cleansed, the wormwood supported the digestion and the oak-bark braced the system.

"What the herbs effected internally, the water effected externally. The thigh douches drew the bad matter together and dispersed it; wading in water and douching the knees not only dispersed matter but acted bracingly on the abdomen and the whole body. Again the action of the back douche was bracing and expelling."

Foot Ulcers

Father Kneipp treated foot ulcers or open sores, with great success. "No illness seems to me more easy to cure than such a disease in the foot," he said. Yet he never actually treated the foot itself. Here is his explanation of this:

"It is quite inconceivable to me that people do not believe that the cause of an open foot is a diseased body, and that to heal the feet, the body must be operated on (with washings). This healing can only take place when all foul matter in the body is dispersed and expelled and the system braced and strengthened ... This is the only natural cure. Nothing should be done to the feet themselves beyond keeping them clean."

It does no good to apply lotions and medicines to force the ulcer to heal over, he said, because this only traps poisonous substances in the body. The ulcer will either break open again, or seek an outlet by erupting elsewhere on the body.

A Reported Case:

A woman, 52, rather stout, had suffered eight years with

a foot ulcer. She had used many salves and medicines and could not heal her foot. Twice doctors had succeeded in healing it, yet within a month, the ulcer broke open again. Father Kneipp told her to use two short bandages (see page 287) dipped in hay-flower water, which was to be warm, during that week. This wrapping was to reach from under the arms to the knees, and to be kept on for an hour and a half. Also, during the week, she was to take two half baths, two thigh douches, a back douche and a whole douche. Internally, she took ½ cup of tea of rosemary, wormwood and dwarf-elder root, twice daily. The pains in the foot diminished on the second day, and from the fourth day on, the feet were quite free of pain.

After 14 days (during which time she continued the applications), she felt absolutely well. The wounds on the feet were smaller. She had an excellent appetite, and was well on her way to being cured. She was now told to take, each week, two back douches, two complete douches and every other day to bind on the abdomen a four-fold cloth dipped in water and vinegar and to keep it on for an hour and a half. Further, she was ordered to drink ½ cup of tea of wormwood, shave-grass and sage daily. After another 14 days, the feet were more than half healed, drainage almost nonexistent.

During the final weeks she was to take three half baths, two complete douches, a short bandage and a thigh douche. And for tea she was now to drink one made of centaury, sage and 10 or 12 crushed juniper berries, ½ cup twice daily, for three weeks. The effect was that both feet healed up, all swelling vanished and her appetite and sleep were excellent.

To insure against further attacks, she continued taking two or three half baths weekly, and at the end of every 14 days a short bandage. Every simple, strengthening food was recommended to her, except coffee, wine and beer. A year later, she was still completely normal.

"In order to make a diseased foot well and keep it so," said Father Kneipp, "fresh air must constantly circulate over it, as I could prove by many examples ... I have been able to bring help and relief in many illnesses, but in no direction have I been so successful as in diseases of the feet; even in those which had been considered past all hope of help and healing..."

Paralysis of the Brain

Father Kneipp used this amazing liquid to treat brain clots or strokes. He said: "When a blood vessel in the brain bursts, it does so from the mass of blood collected in the brain (resulting in paralysis or loss of speech) ... When the seizure occurs, the first thing to do is to draw the blood down from the head to other parts of the body ... To me it is quite incomprehensible how people can lay an ice bag on the head, as it forms an ice wall behind which the blood stops and increases the obstructions.

"My revered predecessor suffered a stroke; he could not speak, his right hand and foot were paralyzed. After laying an ice bag on his head, the blue tint on his face increased from hour to hour ... and the invalid was always trying to tear off the ice bag. At last, the doctor left saying: 'He may last another couple of hours.' On hearing this, I took away the ice bag and wrapped up the feet and also the arms as high as the elbows in clothes which I had dipped in hot water....

"By means of this amazing liquid, in hot soaked cloth, the blood was drawn downward and even after half an hour one could see the blackish blue tint disappearing, and in 12 hours the face had quite its normal color. I kept up the natural warmth ... on the third day, my friend opened his eyes and saw, though he could not speak...

"At midday, I continued the applications and went on from washings, and knee and arm douches, to thigh and back douches. The state of his mind improved, as well as the condition of his body, and even speech came back by degrees, and by the seventh week he began to learn to pray 'Our Father' like the little children. Later he learned the A.B.C. and gradually he came to read.

"He proceeded to Latin and made progress in reading, and later in arithmetic, and in a year he could read the Church service.

"He was now so far recovered that he not only had his full consciousness but was also to a great extent able to think. The speech, too, returned; a little stuttering remained which, however, was of no great importance. He was able to converse ... As his mental and bodily powers increased, we used stronger and more powerful applications. He got to like these very much and found them so necessary that he, himself, managed them daily, although formerly he was not at all in favor of water. The applications consisted of half baths, back douches and complete douches taken in turn."

In describing his treatment, Father Kneipp says: "The best application is daily to wash the whole body three or four times with vinegar and water. Generally on the second or third washing a perspiration appears which is a favorable sign of improvement. As the patient must have all possible rest, his whole body cannot be washed at once; first wash his feet, then his knees and then the upper parts. If the body gets back a little of its activity, wash him all over. Of the head, only the face is to be washed ... The side paralyzed should have the preference and be well washed.

"As the invalid improves from day to day, the arms and feet can be douched and in the following way: the invalid is brought to the edge of the bed so that the foot or arm hangs out over the bed, and then a hose or can full of water is directed over one or both. This douching can be repeated once or twice daily, in addition to washing. The greater the warmth, the more need is there of washing."

Blood must be drawn to the paralyzed parts. "This can best be attained by bandaging the paralyzed parts with a four-fold cloth dipped in hay-flower water four or five times a week. It should be kept on for an hour or an hour and a half ... Besides this the paralyzed parts must either be immersed or douched with cold water each day. One can sit and plunge the whole arm for three or four minutes in a vessel filled with quite cold water. The thigh can also be douched in a sitting posture, but if the patient is able to stand, the effect will be still better. If the invalid be robust, he can apply a whole douche and a special one for the sick part.

"The improvement generally begins in the feet and not till some days later in the arms. There have, however, been cases where the improvement began in the arm and afterwards in the feet." As for food, a simple diet, with no heating drinks, spiced or acid food and absolutely no alcoholic beverages. A spoonful of water every hour assists the bowels. When it is necessary to get them open quickly, said Father Kneipp, boil as much aloes as would lie on the point of a knife with a spoonful of honey and have the person drink a little glassful of it in three or four portions. If the spoonful of water is taken every hour, it is not necessary to take an aperient more than once. A very good effect is obtained by taking black thorn-blossom tea, a spoonful every hour. It is very harmless and works favorably on the bowels, said Father Kneipp. Foods that are not desired should not be eaten.

"I have found," said Father Kneipp, "that several herbs boiled into tea have a remarkable effect; it is as if they strengthened and improved the whole body. Chief among these is tea made of oak-bark, wormwood and juniper berries, which is excellent for the partially paralyzed."

Gout

This simple liquid, water, may bring tremendous relief to arthritis sufferers enabling them to use crippled fingers and limbs once more. It can permanently cure rheumatism and gout, said Father Kneipp. (It can quickly relieve swelling, he said, especially in the hands.) In case after case, feet and legs swollen to twice their normal size were relieved. Foot ulcers vanished. Seemingly hopeless cases were cured.

"Gout in the feet is a malady which frequently appears among people who enjoy alcoholic drinks and eat too much rich food," said Father Kneipp. "This malady usually begins at the feet in the big toe. A burning pain is suddenly experienced ... The joint swells up and the skin is very red. From the great toe the pain goes to the other toes and the whole foot becomes painful. Later on the gout attacks the joints of one or other of the hands ... it attacks the elbow, hip, knee, shoulder and collar bone joints ... suddenly ... the pains disappear ... but the improvement does not last. All at once the pains and swellings begin again and after renewed attacks the swellings harden and form knots especially on the joints of the fingers and this is known as knotty gout...

"It is necessary ... that these swellings should be dissolved and the bad matter expelled ... In curing gout by water ... I used warm baths in combination with cold ones and with douches. I used bandages in order to disperse and dissolve; then I tried bandages dipped in warm hay-flower water and bandages dipped in oat-straw water, and I have with them obtained good results.

"But these applications were always made in combination with cold water, because warm water alone weakens too much and the system cannot so easily throw off the bad matter ... The cure is quickest and surest by the application of cold water." This is the only remedy which cures gout permanently, said Father Kneipp.

Reported Cases:

- "A clergyman came to me," said Father Kneipp. "He had lain in bed for 12 weeks ... and had suffered greatly ... and at the end of the attack he was only laughed at. This made him very angry and he said he wanted to try the water cure. This happened and he was well cured by this amazing liquid; this may have been about 20 years ago. He is now well on in years, and remains cured."

- "A pastor had kept his bed for some time; he suffered very much and had tried all possible remedies without finding relief. I wrapped his feet in a cloth dipped in warm oat-straw water twice a day which was kept on each time for an hour or an hour and a half. The hands which were as painful as the feet I treated in the same way, and had the body washed all over with cold water daily. This last caused a perspiration which carried off the bad matter. After some time the patient considered himself quite cured..."

- "A brewer about 50 years old had gout for many years and was obliged to keep to his bed for some weeks at a time. He feared to take cold water applications alone, and he took during the week two (warm) oat-straw baths ... lasting 10 minutes; then he went for three seconds into cold water, then again into the warm, and so he alternated three times. These applications seemed to dissolve, brace and strengthen and produce perspiration..."

Some of these cases recovered completely. In many, there was a recurrence which was only relieved by this method. "I therefore tried the experiment of using cold water only," said Father Kneipp, "and now I attained quite another result, a result so good that I use only cold applications now in gout except where the patient is very weak.

"Once a stout brewer came to me saying: 'I have suffered from gout for 20 years and for many weeks in the year I have to keep my bed and suffer much pain. As I am well built and otherwise strong I do not want to give up my business, and I wish to make one trial (of the water cure) for I know it is about time for the malady to return and I am anxious if possible to overcome it ... At present I am stiff but without pain.'

"At three o'clock in the afternoon I went with this gentleman into my washhouse and gave him a bracing upper douche and immediately after a knee douche. These did him good and he began to hope. However next morning at eight o'clock, he came with bag and baggage to travel back home directly because his whole arm had swollen seriously and the pain he suffered was almost unbearable.

"I succeeded in persuading him to stay and to douche the swollen arm and the other also very vigorously with (slightly warm) water. The pain yielded during the douching ... In the afternoon about three o'clock he received an upper douche and a thigh douche, whereupon all pain vanished.

"He remained 14 days taking daily two cold douches and he had no more pain. On the contrary the feet and arms were more supple, the limbs more pliable in walking and he was a new man. I gave him instructions on how to make and how to use the applications and advised him to take two half baths, two upper douches and a back douche every week. He followed my instructions from autumn until spring when he came to see me again and said, 'For 20 years I have not had so good a winter. I have an immense business and I can manage it quite alone. Water is golden for people like me.' He is 66 years of age, and since he has tried this water cure (five years) he looks much younger and fresher and declares that for 50 years his work has not seemed so easy to him as now."

For internal use, in gout, Father Kneipp recommended several kinds of tea. First, a tea of mouse-ear (forget-me-not plant), shave-grass and juniper berries for 10 days; then, one of wormwood, knot-grass and juniper berries and tea of centaury, shave-grass and dwarf-elder root. These were taken in very small quantities, 3 or 4 spoonfuls every morning and evening. "If during the cure, sharp pain comes on in the hand, arm or foot, and the joint swells and gets red, the place should be douched for a minute or two," said Father Kneipp. Warm water may be used, but he preferred cold. "The pain will decrease and, if it returns, repeat the douching. As a rule three or four douches suffice and the inflammation passes off," he said.

Amazing Relief for Gravel and Stone

"Among the many evils to which human flesh is heir, gravel and stone diseases may be counted among the worst," said Father Kneipp. "The formation of gravel and stone occurs in the kidney and bladder ... corrupt and unexpelled matter takes refuge in the kidneys and forms little hard crusts ... a reddish sediment is deposited by the urine. When out of this red stuff little grains form in the kidneys, the person is said to be suffering from gravel. The grains of gravel stop for some time in the kidneys, they increase and burn violently but at last may be passed through the ureter ... their passage causes extreme pain. (If they get stuck, there is stoppage of urine.) There are however remedies by which stones, even in the bladder, may be dissolved."

Reported Cases:

- "A gentleman from Hungary who, as he said, had borne untold sufferings for many years and had never been able to find a remedy...tried the water cure," said Father Kneipp. "Now it may have been by chance that just at this time I recommended in a lecture the little herb *knot-grass* specially for gravel and stone. This gentleman immediately collected a large quantity...had the same cooked by his landlady, drank in the course of a few hours 3 cups of this tea, and continued drinking it at his pleasure for several days. After a few hours about 50 rather large stones passed and he felt quite well...This expulsion continued for 10 days, then the passage of small stones ceased.

- "These little stones showed clearly by their shape that they were pieces of larger stones. As no big stones ever passed, I came to the conclusion that this tea decomposed them.

- "As soon as the cure became public property, many people took to drinking this tea out of curiosity, and more than a dozen can show stones that have passed as a result of drinking this tea.

- "I knew a town pastor who for more than 20 years drank every evening a cup of briar-hips tea because he suffered from gravel and stone, and only by this tea was he relieved of pain. He grew so fond of it that he continued to drink it when there was no longer any need to; he certainly had no intention of allowing gravel and stone to come again. He gained his object for he was never ill of kidney disease again and lived to over 80.

- "A gentleman of high rank suffered for years from stone and gravel. In order to get rid of it, he had travelled far and wide and had used many remedies. Still the stones formed and gravel passed daily. We ordered the following applications for him. Weekly, four hip douches, two back douches, three half baths and two upper douches. Daily to drink a cup of tea made of shave-grass, juniper berries and wormwood. After 14 days of this treatment the stones passed in large numbers and the pain disappeared. For the second 14 days he used in the week two half baths, two complete douches, a back douche and a hip douche. By this time he had so far recovered that he could with pleasure follow his profession.

- "A gentleman of about 40 years of age had, according to the doctor's report, stone in the bladder which could only be removed by an operation. He, however, dreaded this operation extremely and all the more because his doctor told him it would be very dangerous. I ordered him, as he was otherwise strong, to take in the week three (warm) baths of oat-straw water ... which were to last 25 minutes and to be immediately followed by a vigorous douche of cold water. We ordered him also to drink 3 large cups of oat-straw tea every day. This treatment continued for two weeks, the stones broke into pieces and so passed off."

"I do not usually prescribe warm baths and would on no account allow weak people to take them; but this gentleman was tolerably strong, and it must be admitted that oat-straw decoctions have a special effect on stone and gravel diseases; indeed they dissolve the stones and carry them off.

"When delicate people suffer from this trouble, it would be well to take two or three warm half baths in the week ... lasting from 15 to 20 minutes. In addition to these there must be applications of cold water, gentle or vigorous as the case may require; for instance, a back douche or half bath daily, and they must drink the tea already named (oat-straw).

"That strongly salted, spiced and heating beverages and food maintain this evil I have no doubt at all. Country people who live nearly entirely on vegetables rarely have gravel or stone diseases; if by chance they do, it is some change they have made in their way of living which is the cause."

Loss of Hair or Baldness

This amazing liquid, water, has been used to stimulate hair growth. "In my opinion," said Father Kneipp, "help is possible in all cases (provided the roots are still alive, and even if only a decayed root remain help may yet be given). Look at a piece of worn out uncultivated land: you cultivate it and bring it into healthy condition and thousands of plants spring up even without anything being sown beforehand. In the same way must the scalp be improved and the hair brought to new growth by helping remedies.

"These curative remedies are first to operate on the system so that it can throw off all bad matter. In the next place one must take care that good blood flows in the system by means of strengthening the diet ... and lastly one must work on the principal part, the head, so that if such living germs exist they may be destroyed. In order to destroy these, I have used for many years a decoction of the common nettle with half-water and half-vinegar and I have made it in the following way: I boil dry, fresh nettles in water and vinegar of equal proportions, the more nettles the better. The decoction should be rather strong, about the same as black coffee. This decoction should be rubbed vigorously into the scalp once a day (for one hour). The rubbing should not, however, take the form of heavy pressure; the pores must not be pressed heavily but gently so that the juice will flow through them. Then the scalp should be washed every morning with cold water in order to remove all impurities. That the hair should be short is a necessity...

"If the skin is not polished, I have never yet had difficulty in reproducing hair ... I have sometimes used burdock root which was held in great esteem by our forefathers ... I have found it good also to rub into the scalp once a week salad Provence oil ... One would scarcely believe how readily the system absorbs this oil. Again, the whole body must be operated on so that it may acquire an equal, natural warmth, a regular circulation and a bracing of the whole system. If a special illness does not exist, it suffices to take two half baths in the week, to wash the upper body three or four times, to walk in water two or three times or to take a knee douche accordingly as the system requires.

"A patient at Worishoffen applied these various things for a few weeks without any result; but a few months later, from his home, he wrote me word that he had then a magnificent growth of hair." Father Kneipp, himself, must have used these methods, for all his life he had a strong growth of hair.

Countless Heart Victims Helped

"There are two prominent diseases of the heart to guard against," said Father Kneipp. "In the first, the heart can degenerate so as not to perform its functions completely as it should, because after inflammation either the valves do not close properly or the muscles become flabby. Sufferers from this form of disease are subject to fever ... the skin has a bluish red tinge, the eyes are dull and tired ... He has pressure and pain about the region of the heart ... short breath, difficulty of breathing, even asthmatic attacks ... such invalids have as a rule cold feet and hands...

"If one desires to cure a patient of heart trouble, one must bear in mind that too much blood exists in the heart and its vicinity because the heart is lacking in strength to send the blood out into all parts of the body ... One must try to reconduct the blood into the feet and hands. If the blood ... circulates freely ... the heart will be in a more healthy condition, its pulsation will be more regular and it will perform its functions with greater ease; the difficult breathing will cease ... headaches will be less frequent...

"I can assure you I have had innumerable sufferers from heart disease under my care and have had the greatest success. This amazing liquid can be used in curing heart disease as follows ... The first thing to be done towards curing heart disease is to get a regular circulation of blood through the body. One must begin gently, but as soon as the body gets strong the applications may be stronger ... the following applications are best: the knee douche, the hip douche and the upper washing. The knee douche or wading in water draws the blood into the feet ... It is also good to immerse the arms in water daily for two or three minutes, by which ... blood is directed into them.

"These applications should be continued for about 10 or 12 days. If during this time a good result has been achieved, pass on to wading in water and back douches and continue the upper washing for another 10 or 12 days. Then for some days longer applications may be made in the form of half baths and back douches followed by hip douches and full douches. The hip douches lead the blood off ... the lightning douche ... would be of great benefit in the second part of the cure. For a person with heart disease the lightning douche must be begun at the feet and continued until they, the knees and thighs, are reddened, a proof that blood is being led into the feet.

"From the legs the douche proceeds to the arms and then for the first time the invalid has the lightning douche on the rest of his body. For people having heart disease, nothing helps more than going barefoot to draw the blood to the feet; they find the tread lighter and the heart quieter. I do not care to use the upper douche for people with heart disease because the stooping is difficult for them and because they dislike it...

"There are ... other maladies known as heart diseases which are quite different from those we have been speaking of. In these the heart is healthy but a fault exists either in the valve or muscles. This causes a palpitation of the heart so great as to render people incapable of action ... In using the water treatment for such ailments the blood must be conducted away from the heart, for such invalids have many bloodless places in the remote parts of the body, owing to the propensity of the blood to linger near the heart..."

Father Kneipp recommended a number of herbal teas in cases of heart trouble. "Bark of oak," he said, "is a strengthening remedy, and if one uses it with wormwood it will be found excellent for the body generally and the stomach in particular. I must, however, specifically warn against taking too much ... only 1 or 2 spoonfuls should be taken morning, noon and night and not a cupful as some desire to drink ... Almost equal to bark of oak in bracing the system are tormentilla and angelica root. There is scarcely a plant or root to be found so good for the blood as tormentilla root. Sage may be used with it. Juniper berries and bark of oak are bracing in their effect on the internal vessels."

Corns

"As a particularly effective remedy for dissolving corns, an old priest recommended ivy leaves to me," said Father Kneipp.

"They were to be crushed and bound on. I have advised this remedy very often with great success. Another good remedy is shave-grass water: boil the grass and dip a piece of linen in the decoction and lay it on; this softens the horny skin so that the scales may be easily removed by the finger."

Varicose Veins Relieved!

For varicose veins, Father Kneipp recommended this amazing liquid, water, as follows: each week, four hip douches, two back douches and two complete douches—for people with a strong constitution. After three weeks, he said the veins get smaller, softer and less painful—at which point he recommended two half baths, a back douche, a hip douche and two upper washings on rising. These were to be taken for three more weeks. To cleanse, purify and assist drainage, he used other Rapid Healing Foods. For example, twice a week before going to bed, he recommended covering the legs from ankles to knees in a cloth dipped in loam water, and twice a week in a cloth dipped in hay-flower water. This assists drainage.

Internally to cleanse and purify, he recommended ½ cup of tea, twice daily, made of shave-grass, dwarf-elder and wormwood, to dissolve and carry off impure matter, which is most evident in the urine. Another tea he recommended was made of tormentilla, rosemary and shave-grass, for the blood. A third tea he gave was of sage, wormwood and angelica root.

Cure of Piles

To relieve hidden piles, which exist deep within the rectum, Father Kneipp recommended wet applications on various parts of the body to draw blood away from the inflamed rectum. Two of these were a short bandage and Spanish mantle (see page 287). Another was known as the foot bandage. This is formed of a one- or two-fold linen cloth, dipped in water, wrung out and wrapped carefully around the foot but not so tight as to prevent free circulation. It should be kept on from one to two hours, but must be renewed at the end of the first hour. He also recommended adding hay-flower or shave-grass to the water used. (Instead of a bandage, a linen sock may be used; dip it in water or hay-flower water and draw it on wet—cover it with a dry sock.)

He also recommended various teas. Perhaps the best of these was one made of wormwood and shave-grass, and another made of dwarf-elder root, juniper berries and knot grass. These helped purify the blood. He also gave a tea made of wormwood, sage and ribwort to improve the stomach. These teas were used alternately, one each week. He told patients to take little or no stimulating beverages and no spiced or strongly seasoned food. The diet should be simple and easily digested. In one reported case, a man with a miserable case of hidden piles, deemed incurable, was cured in six months with this method, without surgery.

Inflammation of the Lungs

Where the lungs are inflamed, to draw the blood away from them, Father Kneipp wrapped the arms and legs in cloths dipped in hot vinegar and water, as hot as the patient could stand it—if the patient felt cold. If the patient felt hot, cold water applications were used on the abdomen. On the chest, itself, a plaster of pot cheese pounded with pot-water to a white ointment was applied. When dry, this was replaced by a new moist application, two or three times, if necessary. This absorbed heat and decreased pain. When the poultice was removed, the patient was washed, after which a healthy perspiration set in. The washings were continued every couple of hours until heat and fever were reduced. If pain returned, another poultice was applied. Do not use ice bags, said Father Kneipp. They are dangerous.

"I have found," said Father Kneipp, "in all inflammatory mischief, especially in inflammation of the lungs, that it is good to take a spoonful of salad oil every morning and evening for three or four days. This oil cools and braces the stomach and protects it from inflammation. For dissolving the mass of mucus which forms in inflammation, I recommend elder-flower, camomile, yarrow, fennel and wormwood. One may make the tea with a separate herb or two or three together. It is of great importance that the diet should be nourishing and digestible and taken in small quantities and that the invalid should breathe good, pure air. Taking every week two or three half baths will keep the system in a healthy, vigorous condition..."

Bleeding of the Nose

"The remedy I have found best is shave-grass tea snuffled up the nose or used as a gargle," said Father Kneipp. The next best thing, he said, was salt water, used the same way, or vinegar. In an extremely difficult case, the patient was not allowed to sleep, despite her drowsiness, as long as bleeding continued. "I made the girl hold her head and ears over a tub and I gave her an upper douche (see page 277) of about 7 quarts of water." The bleeding diminished, and this treatment was continued every day for four days.

Earache and Deafness Relieved!

For discharge from the ear, Father Kneipp recommended water treatments to reduce inflammation—during the week, five or six upper washings, or one upper douche, two half baths and a head douche every second day. Gradually, the discharge will stop, he said. This liquid, in tea form, can be used to cleanse the ear and promote rapid healing: "One may with good effect wash out and syringe the ears daily two or three times with a decoction of shave-grass, or ribwort. The cleaner the injured place is kept the quicker will be the cure."

In cases of deafness, to dissolve obstructions, the head vapor bath was used. A bowl of steaming water was placed so that the patient need only bend his head slightly. A sheet was placed over both head and bowl. Duration: 15 to 20 minutes. Herb water is better than plain water, said Father Kneipp. "There is nothing better than powdered fennel, a teaspoonful of which should be thrown into the boiling water … In addition to the fennel, one may use in the head vapor bath either the yarrow herb, the common nettle, camomile or other good herbs. A handful of any one of these may be thrown into the bath."

When the process of steaming was over, the covering was raised and a shower bath, including the head, was given immediately. Without the shower bath, the patient would scarcely avoid taking a very heavy cold and thus make matters worse, said Father Kneipp. This procedure can dissolve hardened ulcers and abscesses, and open the hearing passages, he said.

Wet packs can also accomplish the same thing, he said: "I could give help to very many by means of herb bandages. A three- or four-fold piece of soft linen is dipped in herb water, bound on the ear for an hour and a half and then removed … Shave-grass tea is of great help also. The decoction is thrown into the ear or a cloth is dipped in it and bound on the ear overnight. Sage is of great benefit when the obstructions produce ulcers. Indeed, all these herb decoctions are good and they are quite harmless to the system." The best method of all, he said, is to douche the whole body, to draw off blood congestion in the head.

Reported Cases:

- A huntsman who, for over two years, had never heard the report of his own gun, came to Father Kneipp, and was given this liquid and other Rapid Healing Foods, which dissolved and removed hardened obstructions in his ears. In a few weeks he completely regained his hearing.

- It may be something as simple as too much wax in the ear. "I knew a woman," said Father Kneipp, "who had completely lost her hearing. The doctor examined the ear and then with a little instrument removed a lot of hardened wax and her hearing was restored."

- A housekeeper had lost her hearing for a long time. During eight weeks she bound on her ear every night a rag dipped in herb water. She had previously applied many remedies without obtaining relief, but the herb water bandage dissolved the hardening so that her hearing was perfectly normal again.

Stitch in the Side

"People often complain of a sudden and severe stitch in the side, in the neighborhood of the lower ribs. Frequently they complain of a burning sensation, extremely difficult breathing, a tendency to vomit and a severe cough which hurts greatly," Father Kneipp observed. "A cloth which has been dipped in water and some vinegar, may be bound to the painful part. After two or three hours it is renewed and generally from one to three such bandages are enough. One may also apply a compress of fenugreek; this operates as quickly as, or even quicker than, a simple water compress.

"If the stitch be the result of hidden gas, then ... soaked hay-flowers, laid quite warm in a cloth or a little bag and if needful renewed in three quarters of an hour, helps the sufferer greatly," said Father Kneipp. "In order to operate internally, one may take a cup of milk in which fennel has been cooked; juniper berries are also an excellent remedy. Tea of bark of oak and juniper berries boiled together strengthens the internal organs; it should however be taken in small portions, about 3 spoonfuls morning and evening."

In cases of pleurisy, Father Kneipp recommended two or three half baths during the week, and washing the body two or three times on arising. He recommended complete rest for a while. The water applications were a mixture of water and vinegar. He recommended teas made of wormwood, juniper berries and shave-grass, and especially tormentilla, as having a good effect internally.

Heartburn Relieved!

Many people experience from time to time a burning, cramping pain and pressure in the pit of the stomach. "A spoonful of weak wormwood tea taken every hour will give help and relief," said Father Kneipp. "The evil will be removed quicker if one mixes the wormwood with shave-grass and sage. Three spoonfuls of angelica-root tea, morning and evening, will also assist in removing the mischief ... A strong and sure remedy for heartburn is the juniper berry cure. Take one day five, the next six, the third seven juniper berries and go on up to 15 and then back again to five...

"Lay on the abdomen a four-fold cloth which has been soaked in water and vinegar, or in hay-flower water for an hour and a half twice or thrice in the week, and the effect will be sure."

Constipation Relieved!

Surprisingly, Father Kneipp found that the best remedy for constipation, was the simplest of all: he said a teaspoon of water every hour opens the bowels quickly, even in severe cases, without straining. This worked remarkably well, especially in cases of stroke, where straining of any kind might be dangerous. He explained:

"This consumption of water causes the food to get into a moist condition and as a douche operates outwardly on the body, so does this spoonful of water act by stimulating the mucous membranes, inciting them to more activity and preventing obstructions."

"Even though the hourly spoonful of water is such an excellent remedy, yet the following external applications must be made; two thigh douches, two back douches, two knee douches and a half bath in the week, which, in a short time, will produce a marked improvement."

Reported Cases:

- One man complained: "For 16 years I have not had my bowels opened once without assistance. I have swallowed much medicine, have undergone massage, but have not been improved one bit. My body is always too full, my head often incapable of thought, my appetite is bad and my sleep is restless." With this liquid, all drugs were discontinued, and in three days his bowels were opened. In 12 days they moved regularly. All his pains vanished, and he could not imagine how his system—which had been out of order so many years—could be cured in so short a time!

- A lady from Munich said: "I had for eight years the greatest trouble with constipation; at length I knew not what to try, for I had swallowed so many things." Then she heard about this method. "It appeared to me quite impossible that a spoonful of water every hour could be of any use. I have daily douched my knees for a minute with water and have done nothing else. In four weeks the whole obstruction in the bowels vanished and now I feel strong and well."

"I advise those who lead a sedentary life to walk," said Father Kneipp. "If there is any warning of constipation, take without delay a spoonful of water every hour, until the bowels are in proper working order. Above all, good nourishment must be provided. I am not against a meat diet but still I think that if meat be eaten at the midday meal with its accompaniments, that is enough, and soup or some farinaceous food is best at night. The food itself should not be heated with many spices and strong seasonings. It is also of great importance to eat good bread. A wholesome, strengthening bread can only be made of a flour which contains all the essential parts of the grain.

"I advise people who suffer much from constipation to take, during the day, between the principal meals, a piece of whole meal bread and about 6 spoonfuls of sugar water; there is scarcely any remedy that helps more towards a regular action of the bowels; and if it is employed for some time, it will increase the blood, expel the gas, get the bowels into order and improve the digestion. I have sometimes advised people to eat during the day a small piece of whole meal bread with an apple, so that the two are mixed in eating. The effect of this is very good if eaten slowly and well-digested. A small portion of whole meal bread, eaten every hour and well-digested, operates the same way. I tried it and was astonished at the effect."

Urinary Troubles

If urination is difficult or painful, it may be due to stones in the bladder, which have found their way to the urethra or outlet. Or the passage of urine may be blocked by swelling caused by inflammation. Another cause of difficulty is cramp produced by a chill, or by drinking a very cold beverage.

> **Stones can be broken up so small that they no longer cause a blockage, said Father Kneipp. This amazing liquid—clean water—is an excellent remedy in the form of baths and teas: two or three warm half baths of oat-straw a week—or sitting baths—lasting about 20 minutes. Two or 3 cups of oat-straw tea should be taken daily as well. Or you can take tea made of shave-grass, briar-hips and juniper berries.**

Inflammations almost always cause swellings. "The best treatment," said Father Kneipp, "is what we use in all catarrhs … to take a complete washing once a day at first, and later twice a day; this will relieve and remove the heat and disperse the blood in all directions. To these complete washings may be added daily two or three compresses or bandages laid on the inflamed spot (soaked in water), renewing each at the end of half an hour." If the patient is strong, said Father Kneipp, he may take a cold half bath—one or two seconds only—daily. A hip douche is excellent, too, he said. Older people may use cold bandages (dipped in tap water and wrung out), to strengthen the abdomen and bladder.

Reported Cases

> • **A patient named Jacob said that if he drank cold beer, he experienced painful urination. Sometimes he could hardly stand it. Father Kneipp made him take a close-stool vapor bath. A handful of shave-grass was put into a bed pan and boiling water was poured over it. He then sat over it for 20 minutes. In a few minutes he perspired freely and urine**

passed while he sat there. On the next day, he received the same treatment, and the difficulty passed completely.

• A patient named Bernard suffered in like manner, but not from the same cause. Neither did his condition yield to the vapor bath, which only relieved him for a time. A cloth dipped in oat-straw water was placed on his back, and another on his abdomen, near the bladder. In 45 minutes, the bandages were renewed and left on another hour. He was also given one-third cup of tea of briar hips and shave-grass three times that day. These treatments relieved him and were repeated, and in three or four days the trouble was gone completely.

Dropsy (Fluid) Drained Away!

Kidney blockage can lead to an accumulation of fluid in tissues in other parts of the body. "In whatever organ the water arises," said Father Kneipp, "this must first be operated on. If the dropsy has it origin, for instance, in the kidneys, they must first be acted upon, and if it spreads itself over the whole body that, in like manner, must be treated. If the dropsy has established itself in the liver, that must be specially treated."

If the dropsy is in the kidneys, a half bath and hip douche will brace, disperse and dissolve, said Father Kneipp. If it has developed in the liver, the best remedy will be wet bandages soaked in tap water and wrung out, applied to the area. The best applications on the whole body are the complete washings, he said, which can be borne by everyone; they cause increase of warmth.

After a few washings perspiration sets in, which is the best thing for the invalid, said Father Kneipp. "Nothing does so much good to the body as cold water, especially if it is mixed with vinegar," he said. "If the patient is still strong, double- or three-fold effect will be produced by stronger applications, such as douches beginning with the simplest and going on to the strongest ... the Spanish mantle (see page 287) will be of great use (if perspiration is not great enough) in opening the pores (use no more than an hour)...

"One can operate internally on the digestive organs and in dissolving and expelling bad matter. The most marked effect is produced by tea of dwarf-elder root, juniper berries and wormwood, and quite a special result by tormentilla root and rosemary. All these herbs, and many others besides, act on the system by dissolving, dispersing, cleaning and bracing."

Dropsy in the Limbs
and Body

Father Kneipp recalled the case of a boy, 17, whose whole body suddenly got bloated. Even his head, hands, arms and feet swelled up. The doctor called it dropsy, an accumulation of fluid in the tissues. All his strength completely vanished, sleep ceased, he couldn't eat and breathing became difficult. He could not urinate, felt ravenously thirsty, constipated and cold. This liquid was applied to his skin in various applications. "On the first and second days," said Father Kneipp, "I made him wash all over four times (then go back to bed each time, under light covers), and at the fourth washing he broke into a gentle perspiration. After this, he had two washings daily. In addition, he wore a shirt soaked in hay-flower water, every second or third day.

"The swelling rapidly decreased, his color became fresher and his normal heat also increased rapidly. Internally I gave him 2 small cups of hemp emulsion daily. Two spoonfuls of hemp seed were pounded, boiled in milk and thus given to the patient. This lessened the heat, decomposed the mucus and carried it off. This was continued for 12 days.

"Then the invalid had a half bath and an upper washing daily; and to improve the stomach, as much powdered angelica root as would lie on the point of a knife was given daily. For diet he had strong broth, grain soup and simple farinaceous food, and meat, such as his system could stand. The invalid was completely cured in three weeks."

In another case, Father Kneipp reported, "A priest, 60, said his whole body was swelling and he was rapidly becoming weaker. A doctor said it was dropsy—accumulation of fluid in the tissues. This liquid was applied to his skin (with a short bandage every other day, see page 287) and other Rapid Healing Foods, including a whole washing of water and vinegar every morning and evening, and a daily drink of one or two small glasses of rosemary wine.

The rosemary wine was prepared as follows: a few twigs of rosemary (green or dried) were cut small, put into a bottle and wine poured over them; when it had stood two days, it might be drunk. When the bottle was empty, wine was once more poured on it; this rosemary wine removes, in a remarkable manner, all the watery stuff through the urine and the action of the bowels.

The priest was once more completely restored to health and able to fulfill his duties after a cure of only a few weeks.

Teeth and Gums Healed!

"I had a bad toothache," Father Kneipp recalled, "and consulted a dentist. He was quite ready and extracted my tooth. Scarcely a couple of months had passed when I had a toothache again, and the dentist took out a second tooth. At the end of a year it was necessary for a third to come out, and I really believe I might have gone on till I had not a tooth left in my head.

"From this I was saved by an old farmer who told me to use this amazing liquid—to hold my head for five minutes under a pipe of running water, declaring that if I did so, the pain would disappear. I followed his advice and succeeded in keeping my tooth. The pain vanished.

"A few years later, I had a toothache again. I sent for the dentist. The answer was that he had taken a glass too much and could not come. In the evening the pain was so great that I sent again begging him to come, but he was unable to do so. It was a cold day and raining fast and as the suffering was great, I waded in the water that stood in the roads for half an hour. From that time to this, I have not had toothache for a single minute."

Father Kneipp told of a young lady whose teeth were so diseased that nine of them were removed. The pain remained and now a fistula, or ulcer, had formed which could not be cured. She had tried every remedy imaginable, yet nothing helped. Reasoning that fistulas on various parts of the body are healed by water, he gave her knee, hip, head and upper douches daily, including a cheek douche (which made the pain cease at once). The ulcer drained profusely. Pain and swelling of the face and jaw dissolved and disappeared. Her teeth and gums were completely healed within a month—by water.

Walking barefoot or on a wet surface often draws the blood down to the feet and relieves a toothache, Father Kneipp observed. Another remedy is figs cut and laid on the gums. Many have been helped by succory, the root of which, fresh or at least damp, is split and laid on the walls of the gums. This root draws out fluid, which reduces swelling, inflammation and pain.

THE PREPARATION OF TEAS

There are many who are not experienced in the preparation of tea and do not know how much of the different sorts one should take to make a cupful. For a cup of tea, said Father Kneipp, one usually takes as much as one can grasp with three fingertips, or, if weighed, nine grains; if several sorts of herbs are to be mixed together, then take for a cup of tea, which for instance consists of a decoction of juniper berries, wormwood and shave-grass, eight or 10 pounded juniper berries, 1 grain of wormwood and 3 grains of shave-grass.

Here are a few more instructions:

- Wormwood must never be taken in large quantities because the tea would otherwise be too bitter.
- If you wish to prepare more than 1 cup of an herbal tea, then take so many times more as you want cups prepared.
- Roots, berries, barks and hard herbal stalks are cooked for a longer period, whereas leaves and blossoms, if they are in dried condition, only have boiling water poured on them; they are then left to get cold, and before being used they are strained.
- Berries and kernels are crushed first, as for example juniper berries, etc.
- If one has bark, blossoms and leaves together to make into tea, one cooks the bark first, then adds the blossoms and leaves, then takes the pot off the fire, covers it up and lets the tea stand 15 minutes, after which it is strained.
- Bark of oak is cooked for five minutes, then elder flowers and strawberry leaves are added and allowed to stand for 15 minutes.
- Crushed juniper berries and shave-grass are cooked together for five minutes, then wormwood is added and the whole again allowed to stand for 15 minutes.

The various curative herbs produce different effects, so that in each illness special herbs make special mixtures which are designed for the relief and cure of a specific malady. For *kidney disease*, Father Kneipp recommended briar hips, juniper, knot-grass or shave-grass, oats and centaury. For *dropsy*, he recommended rosemary, dwarf-elder roots and juniper berries. For disorders of the *stomach*, he recommended wormwood, angelica-root, juniper berries or bark of oak and shave-grass.

THE MEDICINE CHEST

"Everything that I recommend in my medicine chest is easy for poor people to obtain," said Father Kneipp, "for the little herbs grow in God's open air and can be easily collected, dried and made into tea ... It is not always possible to get a doctor at once, and then it is of the greatest advantage to have merely to put your hand in the first drawer of your medicine chest and take out that which is needful to help the sufferer!" (*Note*: most herbs are available at any health food store. If not, ask the dealer to order any you need.)

Father Kneipp recommended the following tea mixtures:

Bark of oak	3 grams	For bleeding, spitting
Tormentilla	3 grams	of blood. Mistletoe is
Cass-weed	3 grams	also very helpful.
Juniper berries, crushed (8 or 10)		Good for diseased
Shave-grass	2 grams	stomach and liver
Wormwood	2 grams	complaints.
Dwarf-elder root	3 grams	Excellent in urinary
Rosemary	3 grams	troubles and valuable
Shave-grass	3 grams	in dropsy.
Elder flower	3 grams	
Dwarf-elder root	3 grams	
Juniper berries (8 to 10 bruised)		For urinary troubles, dropsy.
Centaury	3 grams	
Bogbean	3 grams	Valuable tea for gastric
12 Juniper berries crushed		distress
Ribwort	3 grams	
Coltsfoot	3 grams	For congestion of the
Lungwort	4 grams	lungs or air tubes.

Common nettle......3 grams
Blind nettle.........3 grams   For congestion of the
Mallow flowers......3 grams .....lungs.

Violet leaves........3 grams
St John's Wort ......3 grams   For congestion of the
Watercress..........3 grams .....lungs.

Angelica root ....3 grams
Fennel..............2 grams
Eyebright...........3 grams .....For stomach trouble.

Briar hips ....3 grams
Oat-straw...........7 grams .....For kidney diseases.

Rue ....3 grams
Magnolia root.......3 grams   Good for asthma and
Silver weed ....3 grams .....heart troubles.

Mullein flowers .....3 grams
Elder...............3 grams
Lime-tree blossoms..3 grams .....To cause sweating.

Speedwell..........3 grams   A good tea for de-
Valerian............3 grams .....pression, vertigo, con-
                                     gestion, heart pal-
                                     pitations.

Peppermint ....2 grams
Mullein herb........4 grams   Good for colic or severe
Lime-tree blossom...3 grams .....chills.

Santala.............3 grams   For bleeding of lungs,
Mistletoe ....4 grams .....stomach or severe
                                     bleeding of lower part
                                     of body.

Fennel..............3 grams
Silver weed ....3 grams   Good for cramp,
Rue ....3 grams .....vertigo.

Fennugreek or
Buckthorn..........3 grams
Ribwort ....3 grams   Good for lung
Fennel..............3 grams .....ailments, congestion.

Gentian (either alone or with other
tea), small portion, at most 1 gram,
for it is sharp.................. ....Good for the stomach.

Cowslips and wormwood........... Good for gout.

Pumpkin kernel (25 pieces bruised)
Wormwood........... 1 gram ..... Good for tapeworm.

Fenugreek, or
Sage, or
Shave-grass (as tea, singly or combined) .... Good as gargle

Bilberries, dried and eaten
or made into a tea..................... Good for diarrhea.

"The following make a good tea for purifying the blood," said Father Kneipp, "and one which I specially recommend to invalids with skin eruptions:"

Sage..	1 gram
Rosemary.......................................	1 gram
Yarrow	2 grams
Shave-grass.....................................	2 grams
Juniper berries.................................	3 grams
Ribwort	2 grams
Common nettle..................................	2 grams
St. John's Wort	2 grams
Wormwood......................................	1 gram
Centaury	2 grams

18

Rapid Healing Foods from the Sun for Skin and Hair!

They called him a "crackpot," and neighbors were shocked, when around 1900, Henry Lindlahr, M.D. began treating diseases with sunbathing. Yet Lindlahr had very definite ideas about the healing value of sunshine. He had visited and followed closely the work of the Danish Neils Finsen, who proved beyond any doubt that sunlight could cure cases of tuberculosis of the skin. Later, when Finsen invented the so-called Finsen lamp or artificial sunlamp, Lindlahr bought two of them and put them to use. They were probably the first sunlamps in use in Chicago.

HOPELESS BONE CONDITION CURED!

A nine-year-old girl, with tuberculosis of the left hip and knee, was literally carried to the Lindlahr Sanitarium for treatment. She had been operated upon twice, and had been placed in plaster-of-Paris casts with the prospect of another operation in store. The prognosis was almost hopeless.

Dr. Lindlahr immediately removed the casts, insisting that the affected leg must get sunshine. Almost immediately, the little girl began to improve. The fruit and vegetable diet prescribed might alone have made a tremendous difference, for she had been fed an impossibly rich diet.

As the summer wore on, the little girl took on weight; she grew tanned and beautiful. By September, she was walking—slowly and carefully. By October, the child was entirely cured.

TREATMENT OF PSORIASIS, ACNE, VARICOSE ULCERS!

Dr. Lindlahr had a very definite system of using the sun in healing. Patients were divided into three classes: those that required a sunburn, those that required a suntan and those that required a sunbath.

Patients of the first class were given so strong a sun treatment that their skins almost blistered. The order would be for a "red reaction," which meant an actual sunburn. This was used in certain types of skin eruptions—particularly in psoriasis and acne. It was a command in cases of varicose ulcers. For children with tubercular lymph glands (scrofula, as it was called then), and all types of tuberculosis, sunburn baths were important treatment.

ARTHRITIS, ANEMIA!

Patients with chronic arthritis, or anemia, were given the suntan course. This meant a series of gradual exposures until the patient had a deep, even tan.

The plain sunbath with no particular attempt to get a tan, and with care to avoid a burn, was given as a tonic treatment. It was prescribed especially for convalescents. Dr. Lindlahr was most careful about overtreating with the sun. He held that even as there was a world of good in properly applied sunbaths, there might be danger in overexposure.

LUNG TUBERCULOSIS, DIABETES!

About the first thing he would do in the morning would be to squint at the sun, call for his sunbath schedule, and jot down how long each patient was to stay in the sun that morning. Many patients took only partial baths, browning the legs, the torso or the back. When a particular part of the body was done to a turn, another area would be exposed. This method—now called step-up bathing—was used in cases of lung tuberculosis and diabetes.

PYORRHEA, TONSILS, LOCAL ULCERS!

Patients with pyorrhea were instructed to expose the gums as far as they could to the direct rays of the sun. Dr. Lindlahr had a curved looking glass with which he used to direct spots of sun ray on some local ulcer. He often treated tonsils in this manner. It was all crude, of course—30 years later that same method was being used with special apparatus. But in those days it wasn't done anywhere else in the United States.

Because for us in the temperate zones sunshine is powerful during only three or four months of the year, science has busied itself in an attempt to create substitutes for Nature's gift. We are now besieged with advertisements for all sorts of fish liver oils and their derivatives, sunlamps, irradiated foods and vitamin D concentrates or capsules. Those of us who cannot get sunshine—effective sunshine—should avail ourselves of man-made helps. Children especially need vitamin D. But this vitamin should be used with caution. It is one of several from which we know harm can result from overdoses.

SUNSHINE IS FOOD!

Sunshine is really a food. We know that it makes human life possible through its heat and its creation of vegetable life upon which all animal life depends for sustenance. But we are often ignorant of the fact that either sunshine or some artificial form of vitamin D is directly necessary to the best utilization of food minerals in the human body.

It is not strictly accurate to say that sunshine and vitamin D are identical. What is true is that sunshine, striking the skin, activates certain oils lying just beneath the surface, and the reaction of these oils produces vitamin D in the body. Vitamin D is also released in the system when fish liver oils or other foods containing it are eaten. But sunshine itself has germicidal and healing effects which no vitamin D preparation can duplicate. Even an ultra-violet ray lamp is not a perfect substitute.

To return to sunshine as food, the vitamin D activated under the skin by the sun's rays enables the body to retain and make use of calcium and phosphorus—the minerals essential to formation of sturdy bones, strong teeth and general good health.

Nature has not endowed any ordinary foods with sufficient amounts of this vitamin to be potent. Babies, who are unable to consume those few foods which do contain helpful amounts of vitamin D (egg yolk, butter, cream, cheese and certain sea foods), need the certain protection of fish liver oils. Normal, healthy adults can probably meet their needs in winter months by eating enough of the common foods listed above, and availing themselves of all natural sunshine possible. Sunlamp treatment helps.

SUNOIL AND SUNWATER!

No one in those early days knew that any such substance as vitamin D existed. That plants or living substances could store actual sunlight in the form of vitamin D was not to be understood for many years to come. Dr. Lindlahr was putting this principle to work almost 30 years before it was discovered—with sunbaths and the use of sunoil and sunwater.

All the olive oil used in salad dressings at the Sanitarium was exposed to the sunlight in flat-bottomed dishes for an hour or two before it was served. The kitchen help used to shake their heads over this custom. They thought it was crazy. But the fact remains that the olive oil gathered potency in vitamin D—long before anyone knew the whys and wherefores (just as Scandinavian mothers have fed their children cod liver oil in winter months for centuries, unaware of its vitamin content).

VARICOSE ULCERS HEALED!

In 1916, Dr. Lindlahr proved that his prized sunoil had unmistakable virtues by an interesting experiment. One afternoon, his son, Victor, who was a medical student, heard some patients discussing the sunoil. One said: "It's nothing but olive oil that the doctor soaks in the sun." Young Lindlahr had quite a discussion with his father about it. "It's making you seem ridiculous," he said. "But it works," said Dr. Lindlahr. "I'll show you."

About a week later, Dr. Lindlahr showed his son a case: a waiter who had two running ulcers due to varicose veins, one on each leg. The one on the right leg was about a quarter of an inch in diameter. The one on the left leg was fully an inch and a half wide. It had been running for almost two and a half years.

This was in the latter part of October when the sunbaths were closed. Dr. Lindlahr handed him two bottles—brown bottles that held about 16 ounces of fluid. The red-labeled bottle contained ordinary olive oil, and was marked, "For the right leg." The white-labeled bottle contained olive oil that Dr. Lindlahr had sunned, and read, "For the left leg." The patient was instructed to dab the respective oils over the entire area of each sore and about half of the affected legs.

Four weeks later, to the day. Dr. Lindlahr called his son into the office again and had the patient show his legs. The ulcer on the left leg was completely healed. The ulcer on the right leg was still open—healing gradually. Dr. Lindlahr smiled. "You see what the sunoil does?"

As his son recalled, "There was no question but that the ugly left-leg ulcer had healed beautifully. Father told the patient to use the white-labeled bottle on the right leg. Within a week the little ulcer was entirely healed.

"Father's sunoil was a vitamin D product. Today, in medical circles, white Vaseline is fortified with vitamin D, and cod liver oil is used on wounds because of the healing effect of the vitamin D and A that it contains."

SKIN AND LUNG INFECTIONS, ARTHRITIS AND RHEUMATISM OFTEN CURED!

Sunshine's virtue as a calcium-holder and builder of bones is thus not its only important recommendation. Antiseptic and therapeutic effects are produced by the action of the sun's rays on bare flesh. Skin infections, major and minor, lung trouble, streptococci infections, rheumatic fever and arthritis or rheumatism are all benefited—often cured—by the effects of nothing more than direct sunshine, said Dr. Lindlahr, Jr. Plus, of course, the requirements of fresh air, rest, proper food and other natural measures. These last-named alone, however, would not be enough; sunshine is a specific for at least a dozen diseases.

PREPARING SUNWATER

Every morning that the sun shone, Dr. Lindlahr used to have what he called sunwater prepared for his patients. This was water which had been exposed to the direct rays of the sun. A big flat earthenware tub was used for the purpose, and the water was stirred in the morning sunshine. Then it was poured into big pitchers, and as Dr. Lindlahr made calls from room to room, patients he thought needed sunwater were given a glassful to drink right then and there.

FOR ULCERS, STOMACH AND INTESTINAL INFECTIONS

He insisted particularly that all individuals with stomach and intestinal infections or ulcers must have the water. They drank it gratefully. Many of them didn't know what it was—just thought it was medicine of some kind.

There is a classical experiment which proves that certain forms of matter, including water, can be endowed with antiseptic and germicidal power. Water cannot be impregnated with vitamin D (some form of fat is needed before a substance can be made to hold this vitamin) but it can absorb germ-killing power.

Researchers found, for example, that water containing typhoid germs could be made safe if it were spread in a shallow pan and placed in strong sunlight for a period of time. They discovered, too, that chemically pure water which has been exposed to the sun, bottled and stored, will not play host to similar germs. The invaders will die. With this knowledge of the sun's power, everyone should make the most of this free gift of Nature.

WHAT YOU SHOULD KNOW ABOUT SUNBATHING!

In lieu of sunbathing at the beach, rooftops, fire-escapes and front lawns should be utilized—windows can be thrown up to admit unhampered light (ordinary window glass removes ultra-violet rays).

It should be clearly understood that too much sun can be almost as destructive as no sun at all. Regard sunshine as food. No one would dream of eating an elephant's meal one day and going without food for weeks or months. Yet city people sometimes spend hours at a blazing beach in July—and never see the sun again until many weeks later. An occasional day at the shore or a two-week sunburning while on vacation may be extremely painful and certainly does not substitute for daily exposures.

A STEP-BY-STEP METHOD!

The proper technique of sunbathing is still that which Dr. Lindlahr insisted upon for his Sanitarium patients more than 50 years ago. Begin gradually, tan the entire body evenly and then use common sense about remaining too long in bright sunshine. Children and adults with light, easily burned complexions, need to be particularly careful.

For the average adult who is neither especially blond nor dark, the following method was suggested by Dr. Lindlahr, Jr. Take your bath between the hours of eleven o'clock in the morning and two o'clock in the afternoon. This is the period of the sun's greatest strength, and it is the time when the sun best penetrates air pollution, such as smoke, dust and dirt. In open country, the best hours are earlier in the morning or later in the afternoon.

DAY 1—Keep the head covered but remove all other clothes if privacy is possible. If something must be worn, choose white, loosely-woven cottons, and wear no more than necessary. Lie face down for five minutes. Then leave the sunlight for a minute or two and rest.

Return and lie on the right side for five minutes. Take another short rest, then go back to the sun and lie on the left side for five minutes. Rest again, and finish with a five-minute interval in the sun while lying on the back.

After the sunbath is completed, the pores are open and there has been a heat loss from the body. Readjust your circulation and prevent loss of energy by taking a cold sponge bath. This practice, and that of taking a short rest between exposures, must not be neglected. They enhance the value of the sunbath.

DAY 2—On the second day, the time duration for each position can be increased three minutes. Make a similar increase each day until the fourth or fifth day. That would mean, on the fifth day, that each side of the body would be receiving approximately 17 minutes of direct sunshine. Up to 20 minutes is safe.

When you have a complete tan, you will be reasonably safe from burning, but common sense should tell you that long exposures are neither healthful nor necessary. They do nothing but thicken and darken the skin—Nature's way of shutting out unneeded sunshine—so that the system fails to benefit.

ACCOUNTING FOR VARIATIONS IN SKIN COLOR!

Special cautions should be observed by extremely blonde individuals or those who have naturally sensitive skins. In their cases, the time for beginning exposure of each side of the body should be reduced to two and one-half minutes (exactly half) and should be increased at half the normal rate—one and one-half minutes—each day. People who can't tan, who just burn, should cut even these exposure times to an amount safe for their skins, and take the baths oftener to make up for the loss.

Red-headed people who freckle or burn easily should follow the rules for blondes. The other type, with less sensitive skin, is able to stand the regular routine.

The deeper the natural color of the skin, the longer the sunbath must be for good effects. Black people require very long baths because their pigmented skin shuts out most of the sun's rays.

SUNBATHING INFANTS

Babies and children need sunbaths even more than adults, but their tender, sensitive skins must be treated with care. Never make the mistake of introducing a baby or a young child to the sun with a full body bath. Babies should begin with very small doses of sunshine. Expose the legs the first day for only a minute, if in the country or semi-rural areas, and two minutes if in a city where the atmosphere is not clear. The arms may be similarly exposed the second day, the back the third. Increases in time must be made very slowly, and the head and eyes protected at all times.

SUNBATHING CHILDREN

The average child past two years of age may begin with a three-minute exposure on each side. The rests must be observed between each exposure. Increase the time by two minutes a day until the child is receiving 15 minutes' exposure on each side of the body. Continue at this level until the skin is safely tanned.

It is important to remember, of course, that children vary just as do adults. The extremely fair child and the redhead must have only half the normal beginning sunshine, and increase their time in the sun at half the normal rate. Very dark children may start with longer periods and increase them more rapidly.

Because children are outdoors so much in the summer, they are more apt than grownups to get an overdose of sunshine. If the child shows such symptoms as a blotchy skin, fitful sleep, irritability and loss of appetite, it is quite possible that he has been permitted to play in strong sunshine too long.

USING SUNOILS!

When these routines are followed, the normal individual should have no need for a sunburn preventive or a sunburn soother. But sensitive people, who know they are going to be exposed for a longer time than their skins will comfortably permit, should protect themselves before and frequently during exposure with some form of suntan oil. Old-fashioned cocoanut and castor oils are excellent.

TREATING SUNBURNS!

Bad sunburn, like any burn, should be treated by a physician. Freshly brewed tea, strained and cooled, is both comforting and healing to the ordinary case of sunburn, said Dr. Lindlahr, and commercial creams, oils and pastes can be bought anywhere. The tea is effective, said Dr. Lindlahr, because of its content of tannic acid—a solution of which has been used as treatment for even the most severe burns.

SPECIFIC USES OF SUNLIGHT
IN TREATING VARIOUS AILMENTS!

Victor Lindlahr, M.D., who carried on his father's work, stated: "I can testify from first-hand experience that hundreds and hundreds of cures of various ailments were made at the Sanitarium over a period of many years with only natural sunlight (actinic therapy). Patients just sat in the sun and exposed injured parts to its healing rays until they developed pinkness (first degree exposure), redness (second degree exposure) or tan, as the case might be...

"The most spectacular effects of sunlight are observed in some of the skin diseases. For many of them, notably lupus or tuberculosis of the skin, sunlight is a specific. In most of these cases, it is desirable to treat not only the affected area but also the body generally. Sun burning of the place where the lesion exists is usually advised." Dr. Lindlahr listed the following treatments:

Acne, Pimples

"Although acne is basically due to certain body chemistry disturbances based upon dietary errors, and is complicated by constipation, allergy and other factors, the local effects of sunlight upon acne are extremely beneficial, particularly when the disease has progressed to the stage of infection.

"The affected portions of the skin should be exposed to the sun's rays until an actual sunburn is attained. (Before a treatment is begun, matter should be gently squeezed from any blackheads which may be present.) Then it is better to cease exposures until the sunburn has subsided, when another effective burn can be received. Technically, these burns are called erythema solare (diffuse redness caused by sunlight).

"One of the beneficial effects of the burn is that the diseased skin peels off and is replaced by hardier cells. Also, the sunburn brings a congestion of blood (hyperemia) to the affected area. Those parts of the skin which are not afflicted with acne should be covered.

Baldness

"There are various types of baldness, of course, but the general creeping baldness which afflicts so many men can often be stayed and growth of new hair stimulated by sunlight. Sunlight sufficient to produce a pinkness or redness of the skin helps to nourish hair roots. Allow the scalp color to fade after each treatment before using sunlight to secure another pink reaction. All other parts of the body should be covered so that the stimulating effect of the sunlight may be concentrated on the scalp.

Red Nose, Boils, Poison Oak or Ivy, Shingles, Lupus (TB) of the Skin, Birthmark, Fingernail Inflammation, Chilblains, Barber's Itch

"*Red nose, whisky nose, acne rosacea,* may be treated with gentle sunlight exposures (just long enough to produce a slight pinkness) once or twice a day until the affected area is tanned. In case of *boils, furuncles, carbuncles,* sunlight exposure to the extent of producing a burn may abort or cure any of these infections. Cover the rest of the body, exposing only the affected tissues. *Poison ivy and poison oak* are benefited by erythema doses. Spreading is usually checked. *Shingles* are greatly helped by erythema doses. Sunlight is specific for *lupus (T.B.) of the skin,* but treatment should not be undertaken without the supervision of a physician trained in the proper technique. Certain types of *birthmarks* respond beautifully to sunlight, but here, too, it would be wise to have skilled supervision. *Inflammation of the fingernails* responds remarkably to erythema doses. For *chilblains,* erythema is often a cure and usually prevents recurrence. *Barber's itch* is definitely benefited by sunlight.

Psoriasis

"While psoriasis is a disorder probably due to derangement of the body's fat metabolism and is treated primarily with fat-free diet, erythema and general sunlight are extremely helpful locally.

Pruritis

"This intolerable itching, especially when it affects the pelvic parts, is most often due to the presence of molds, somewhat similar to those that produce athlete's foot. Exposure of the affected parts to sunlight to the extent of erythema is quite helpful.

High Blood Pressure

"A gradually acquired suntan is most beneficial in cases of high blood pressure. Perhaps the dilation of surface blood vessels is the chief factor, or it may be that certain metabolic changes are brought about by sunlight. At any rate, the acquiring of a suntan is an excellent adjunct to the regular treatment of high blood pressure. However, abrupt or severe sunburn is apt to heighten the blood pressure."

Other Ailments Helped!

According to Dr. Lindlahr, suntan seems to be of specific benefit in the following cases: 1) menstrual disturbances, 2) bronchial asthma, 3) so-called neurasthenia or nervous diseases, 4) chronic arthritis, 5) sciatica, 6) lumbago, 7) bone fractures, 8) tuberculosis (very gradual exposures), 9) allergic disorders, 10) chronic catarrh, 11) sinus troubles, 12) pyorrhea, 13) rickets.